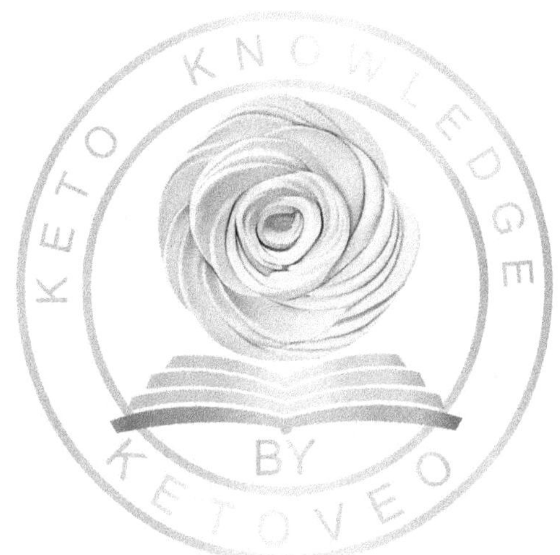

Go to **www.ketoveo.com** for more guides and resources to help you on your keto journey.

Contents

Basic Stretches Everyone Should Know   87

At Home Full Body Workouts

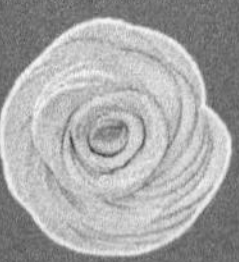

How to do Calf-Raises

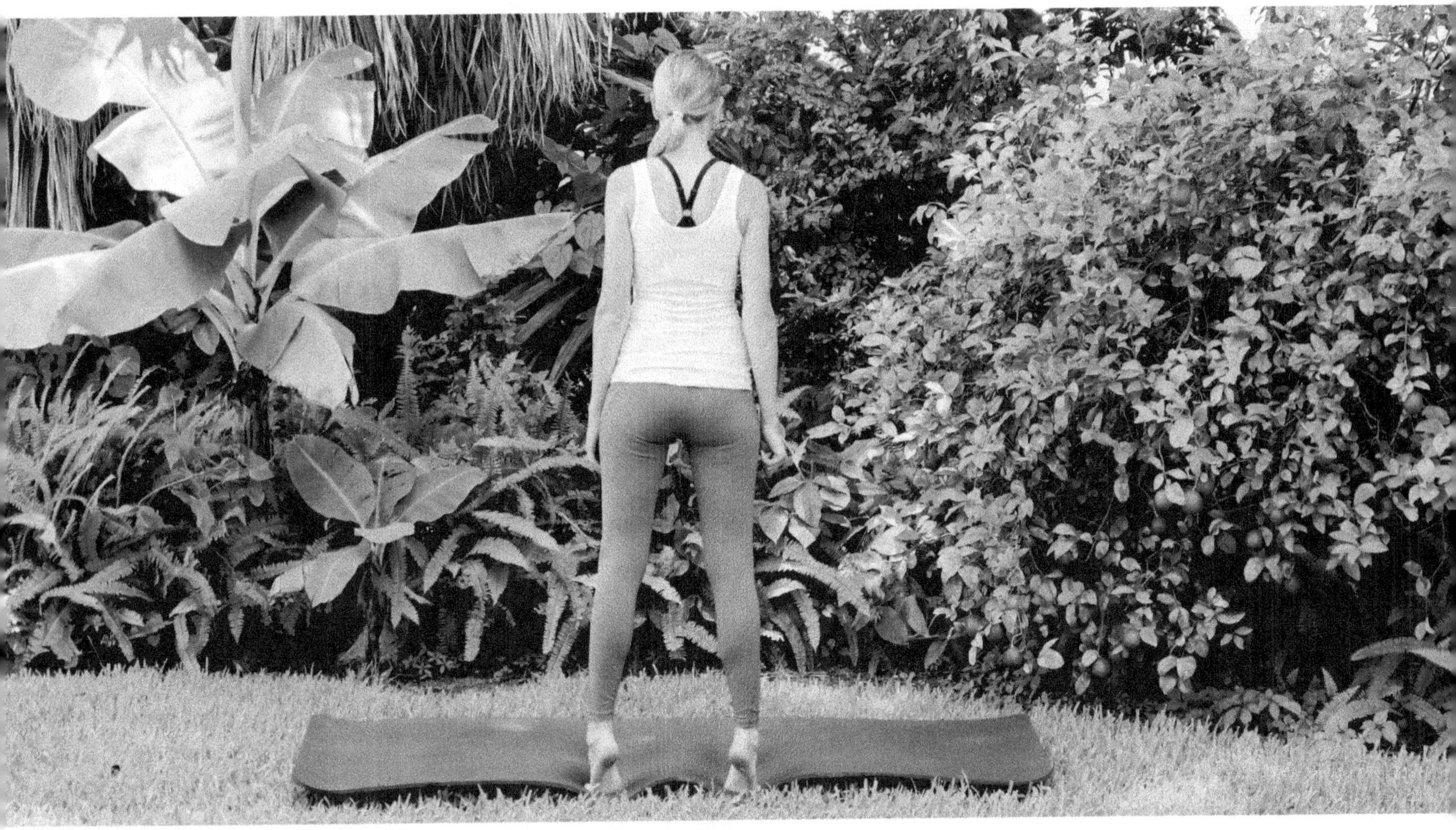

1. *Get into a standing position, slowly rise up onto your toes, keeping the knees straight and heels off the floor.*

2. *Hold briefly, then come back down.*

3. *Repeat.*

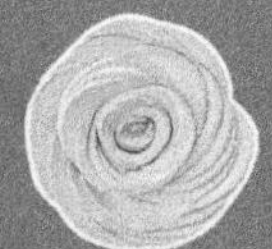

How to do Sumo Squats

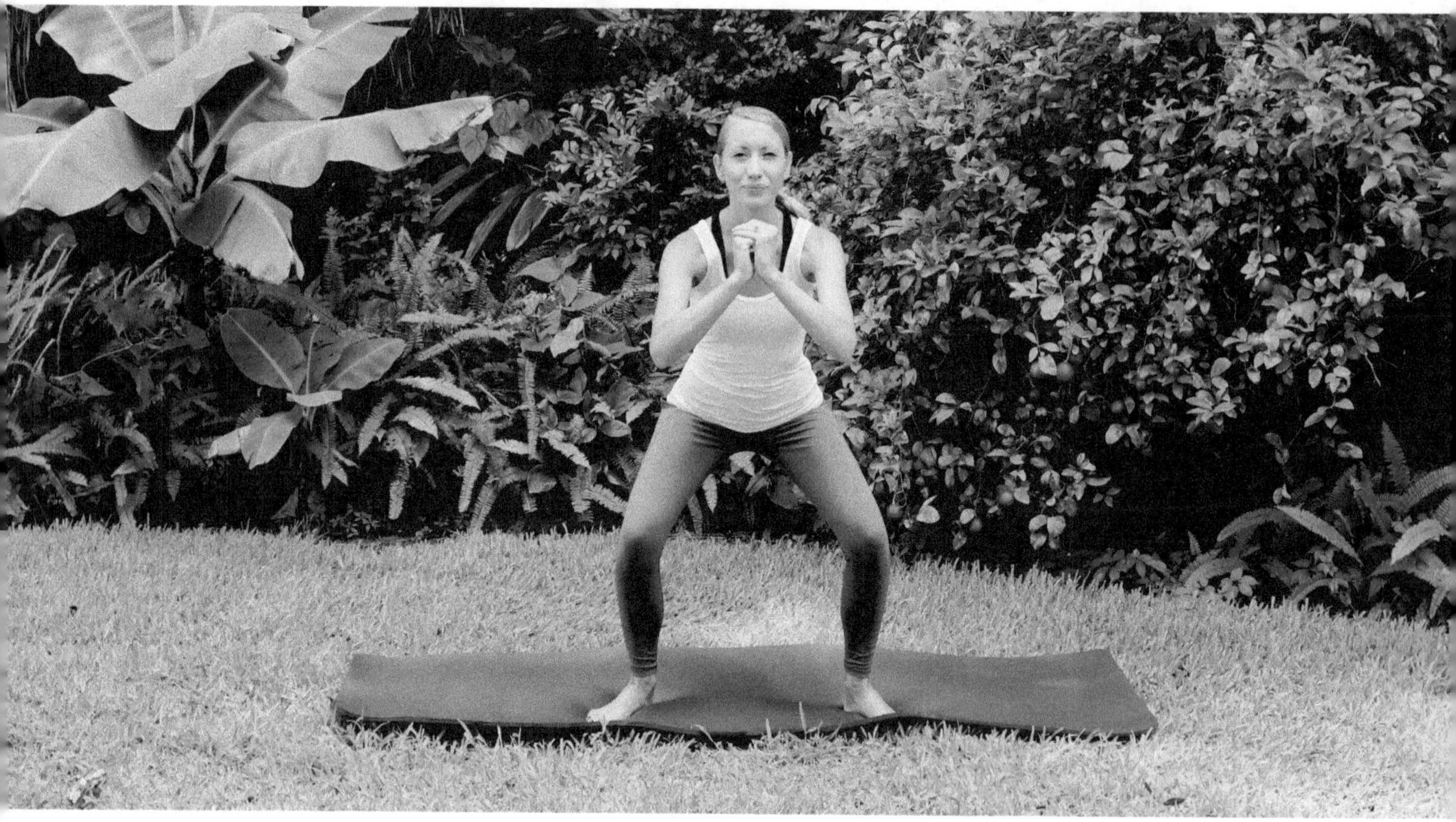

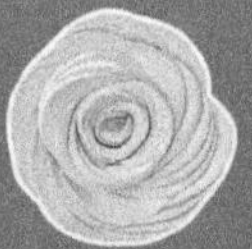

1. *Take a very wide stance and place your palms together in front of you.*

2. *Begin the squat by sitting back, and focussing on keeping your chest up and knees pushed out.*

3. *Repeat.*

How to do Air Squats

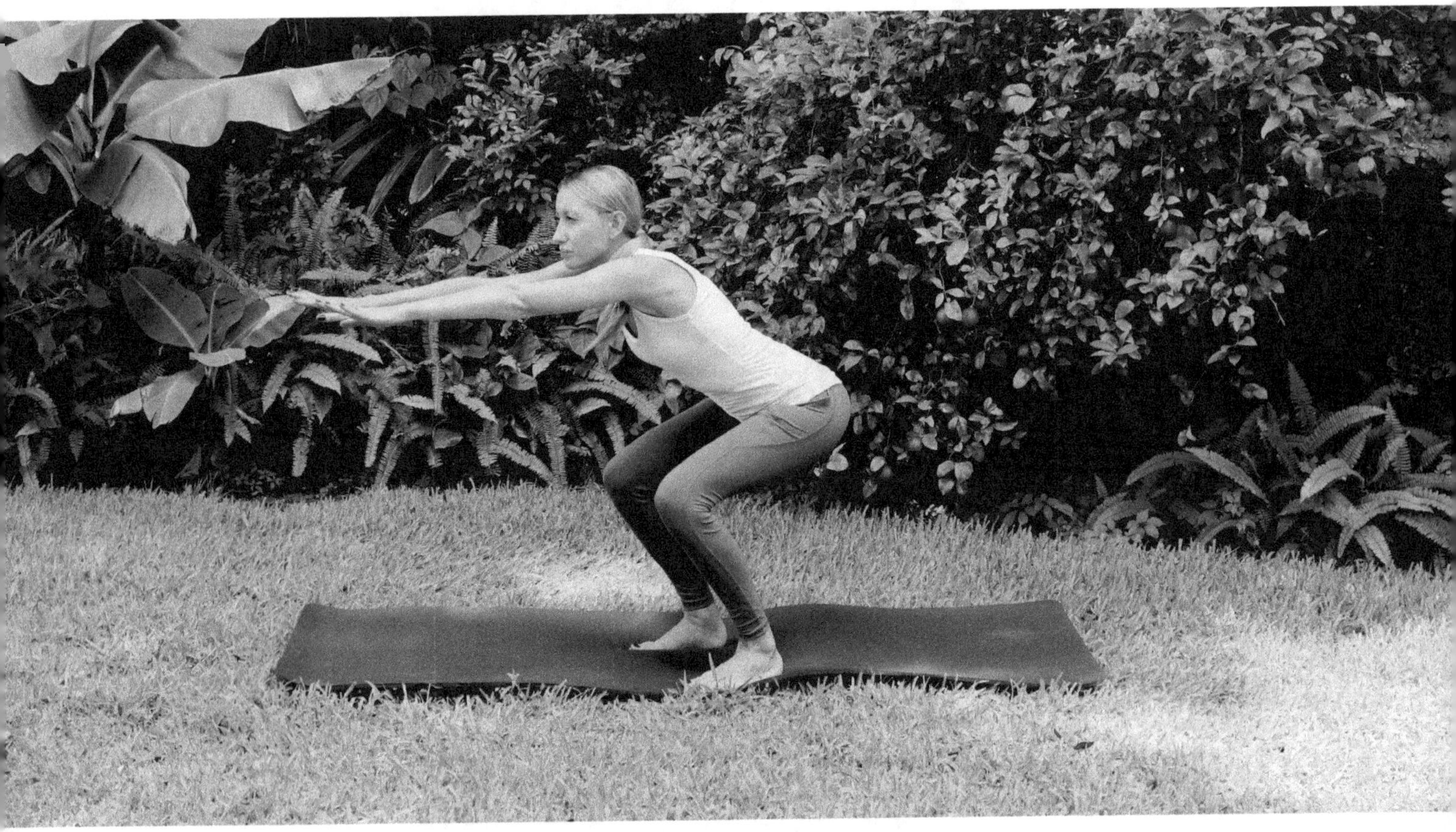

1. *Stand with your feet hip-width apart and your feet facing forward. Slowly sit back by bending the hips and knees until your thighs are parallel to the floor.*

2. *Keep your weight on your heels throughout the movement and press through them to return to a standing position.*

3. *Repeat.*

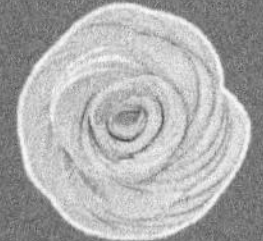

How to do Static Lunges

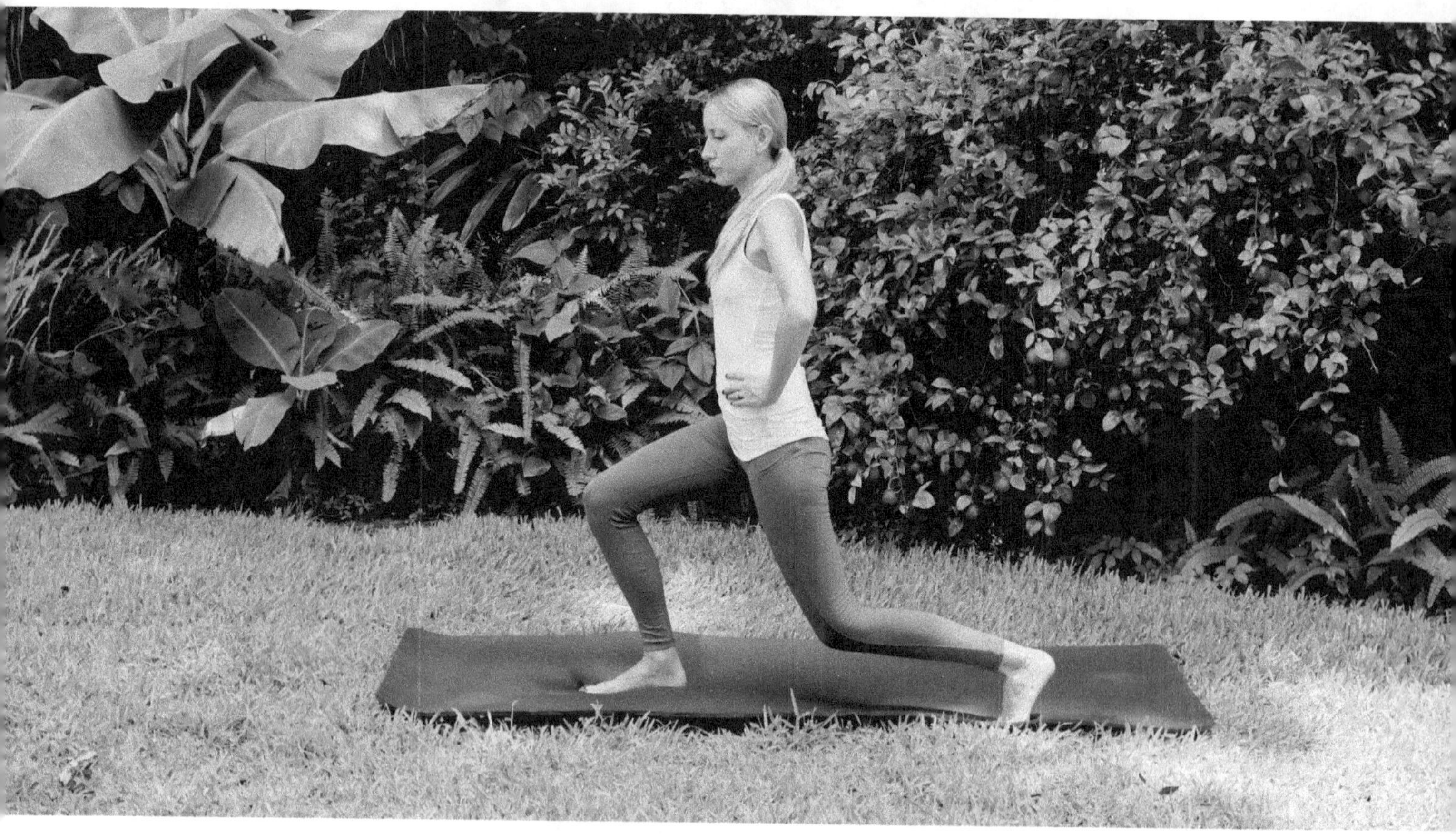

1. Stand with your hands on your hips and take a long stride forward. Your feet will stay in this position throughout the exercise.

2. Slowly lower your body until the knee of your opposite leg is close to or touching the floor.

3. Push back up into the starting position and repeat with your opposite leg.

www.ketoveo.com

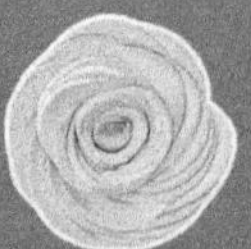

How to do Reverse Lunges

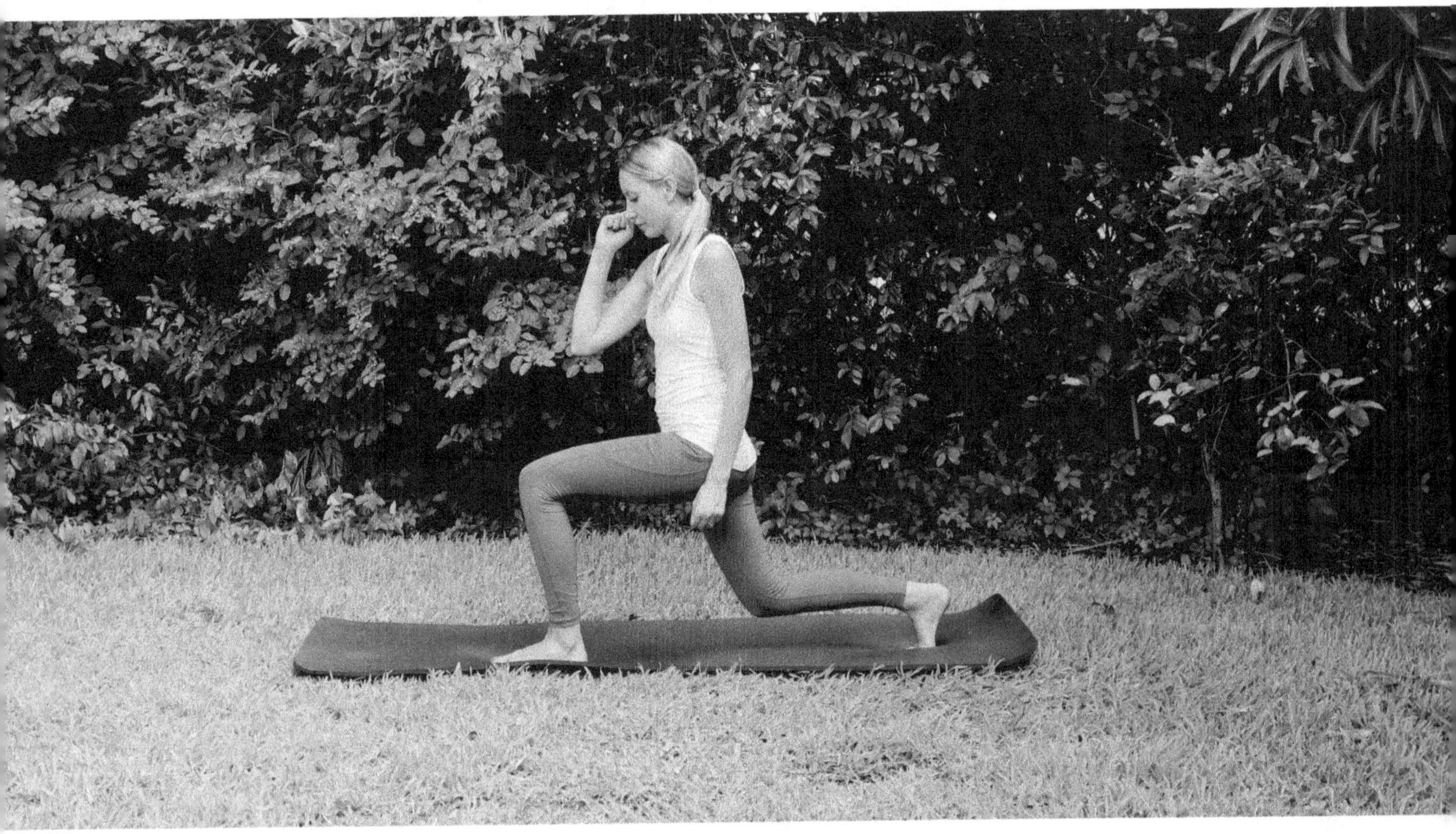

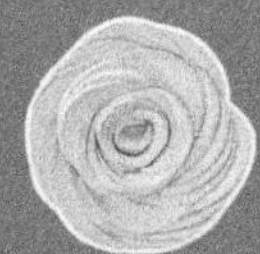

1. *From a standing position take a wide step back and slowly lower your body until your back knee is close or touching the floor.*

2. *Push back to starting position and repeat with your opposite leg.*

How to do Bulgarian Split Squats

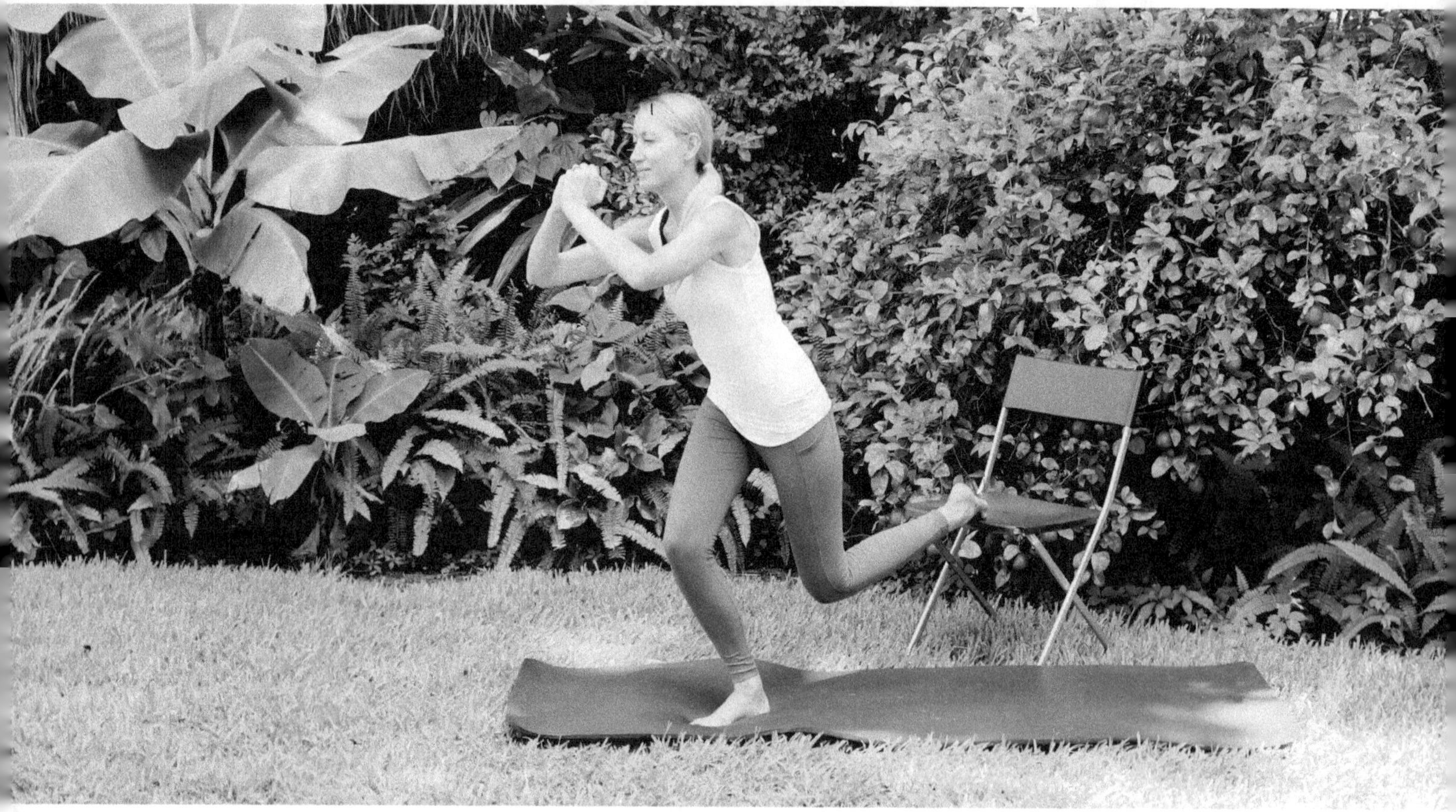

1. Stand with your back in front of a raised surface and place one foot behind you on top of the raised surface.

2. Keeping your torso upright, descend until the knee of your rear leg touches the ground, and then push back up to return to the starting position.

3. Make sure the knee of your front leg doesn't move past the toes.

4. Repeat and alternate legs.

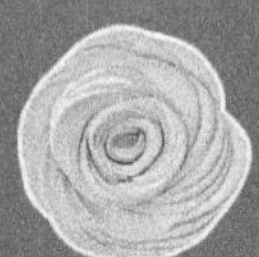

How to do Glute Bridges

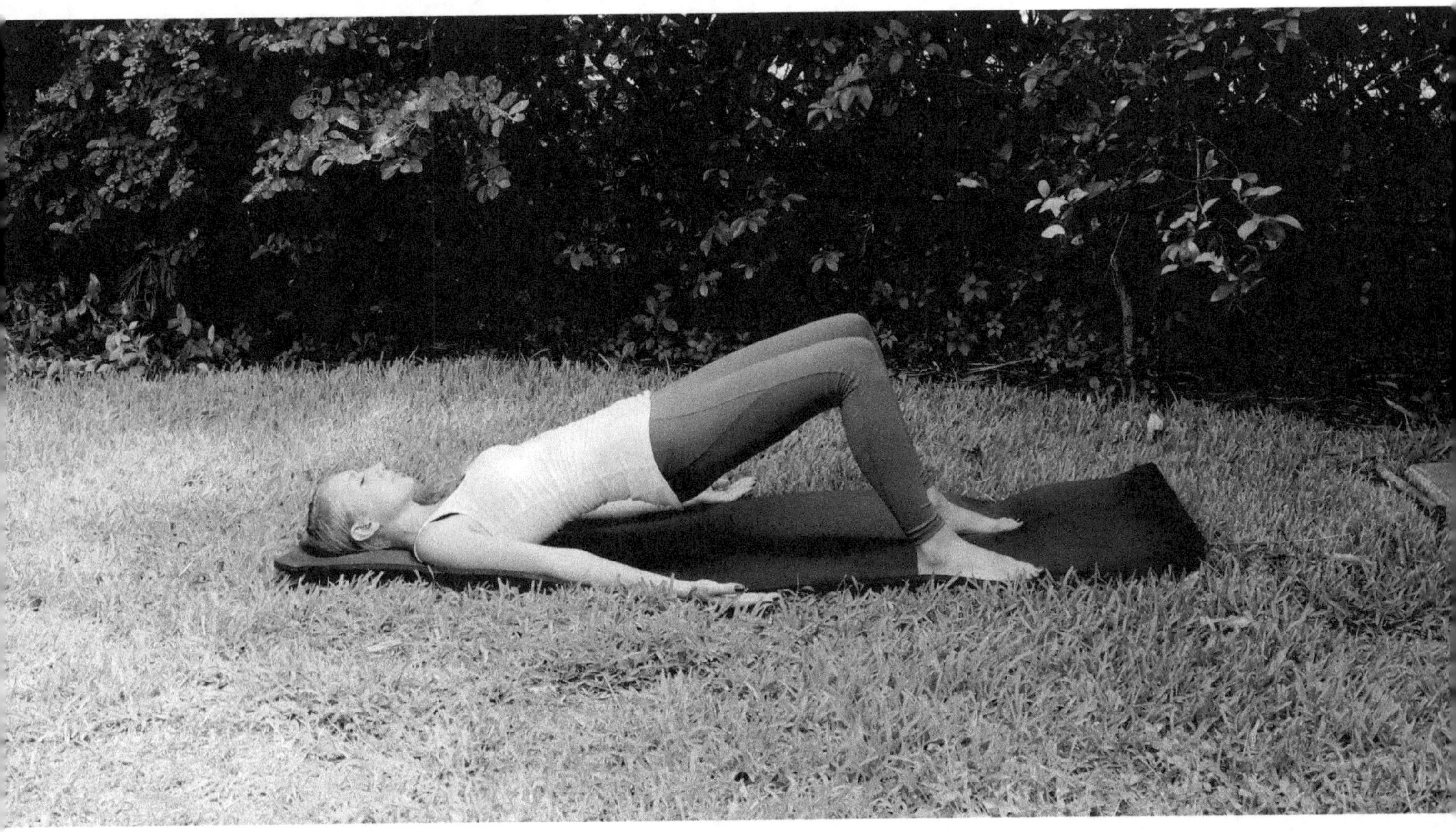

1. Lie on your back with your knees bent at 90 degrees and your hands at your sides.

2. Push through your heels and use your glutes to lift your hips as high as possible.

3. Pause at the top and slowly return to the starting position.

4. Repeat.

How to do Side Lying Clams

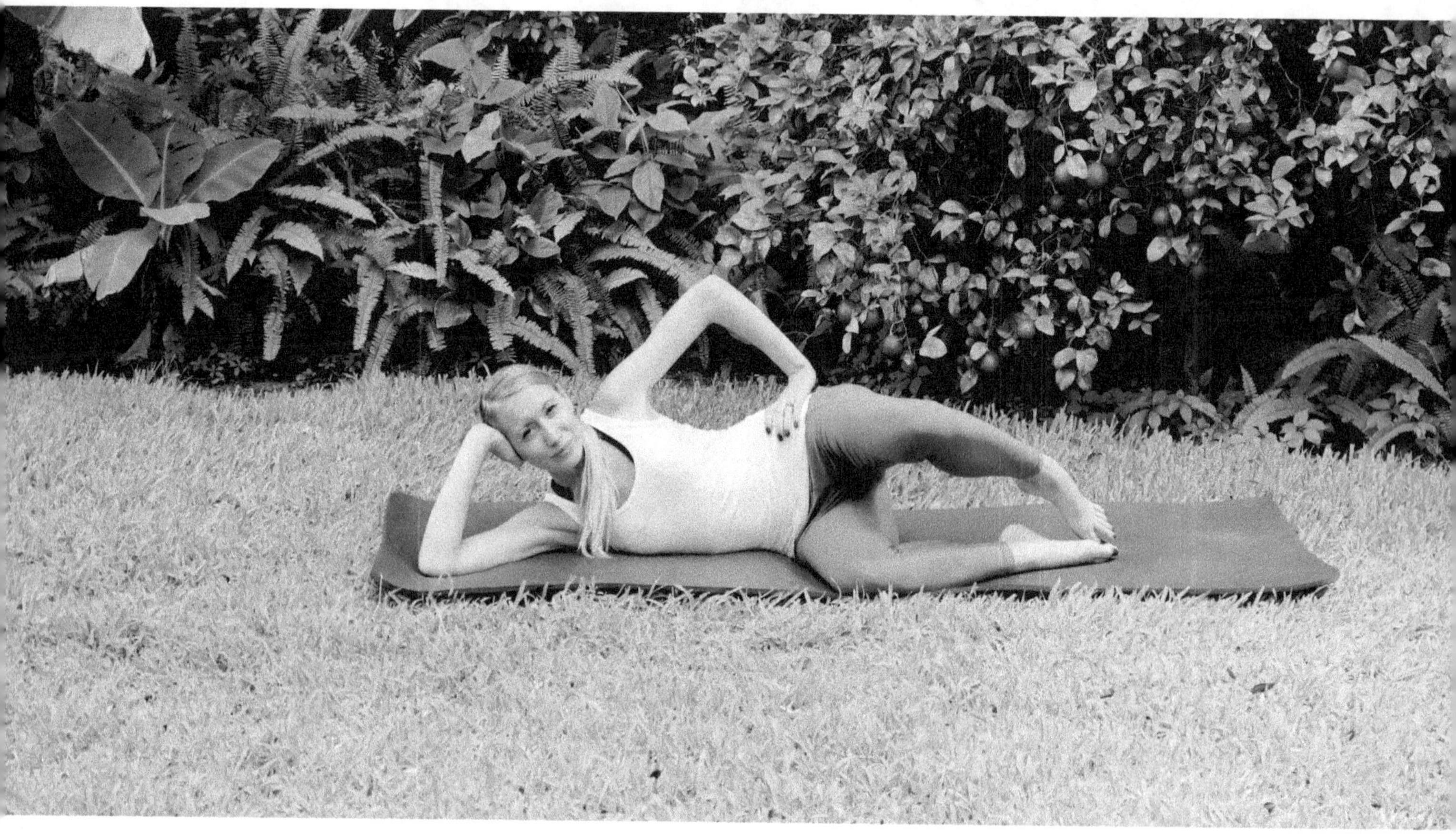

1. Lie on your side with your knees bent at 90 degrees and heels touching each other.

2. Open your knees by flexing your glutes and hold the position. Slowly return to the starting position.

3. Repeat and alternate sides.

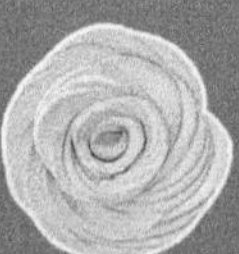

How to do Donkey Kicks

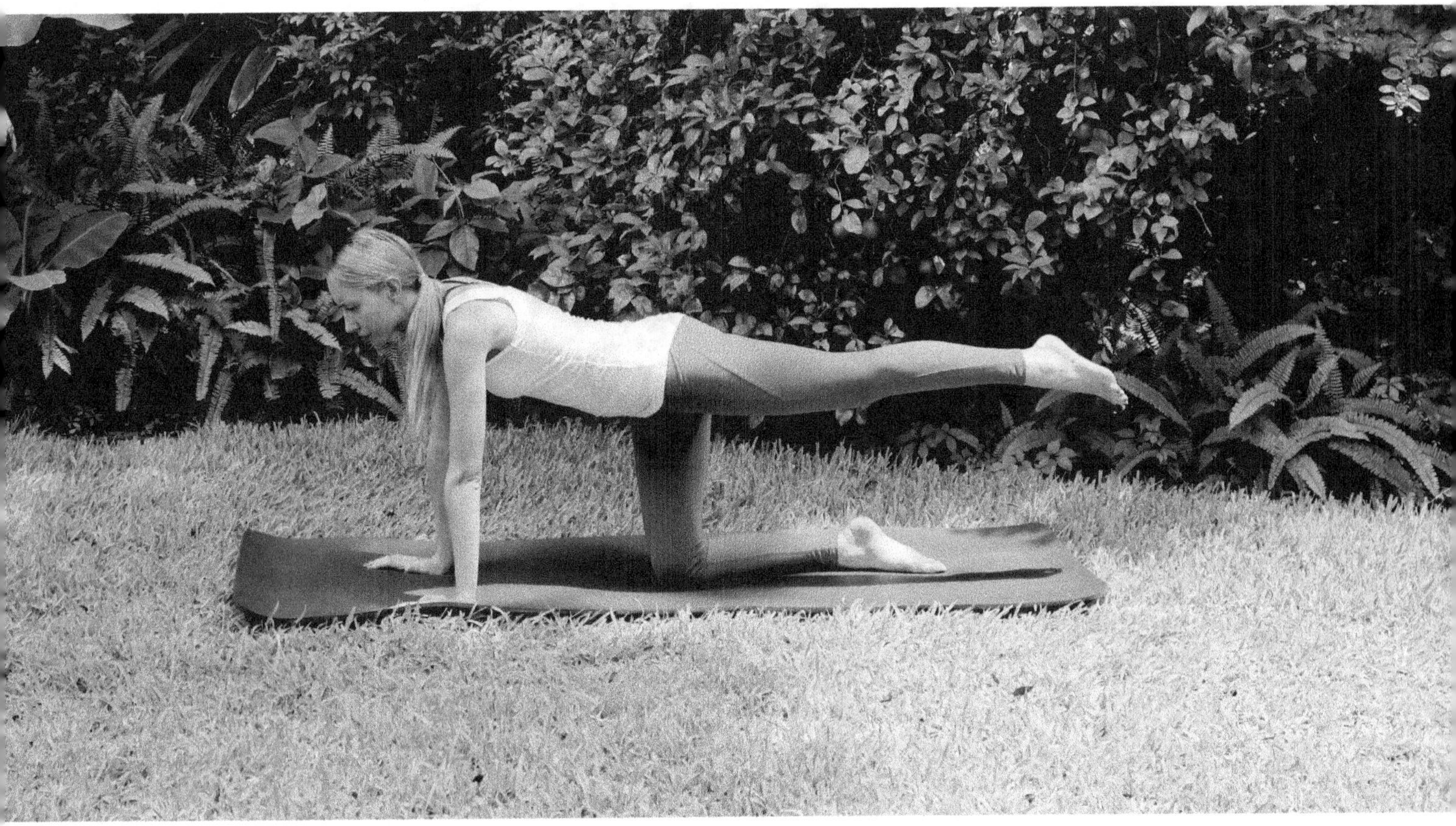

1. *Get down on all fours with your back flat.*

2. *Kick one leg until it is straight behind you and slowly return to the starting position.*

3. *Repeat with the opposite leg.*

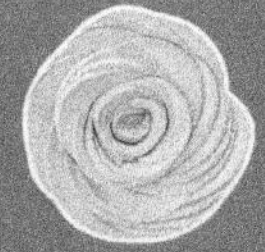

How to do Bent-Leg Donkey Kicks

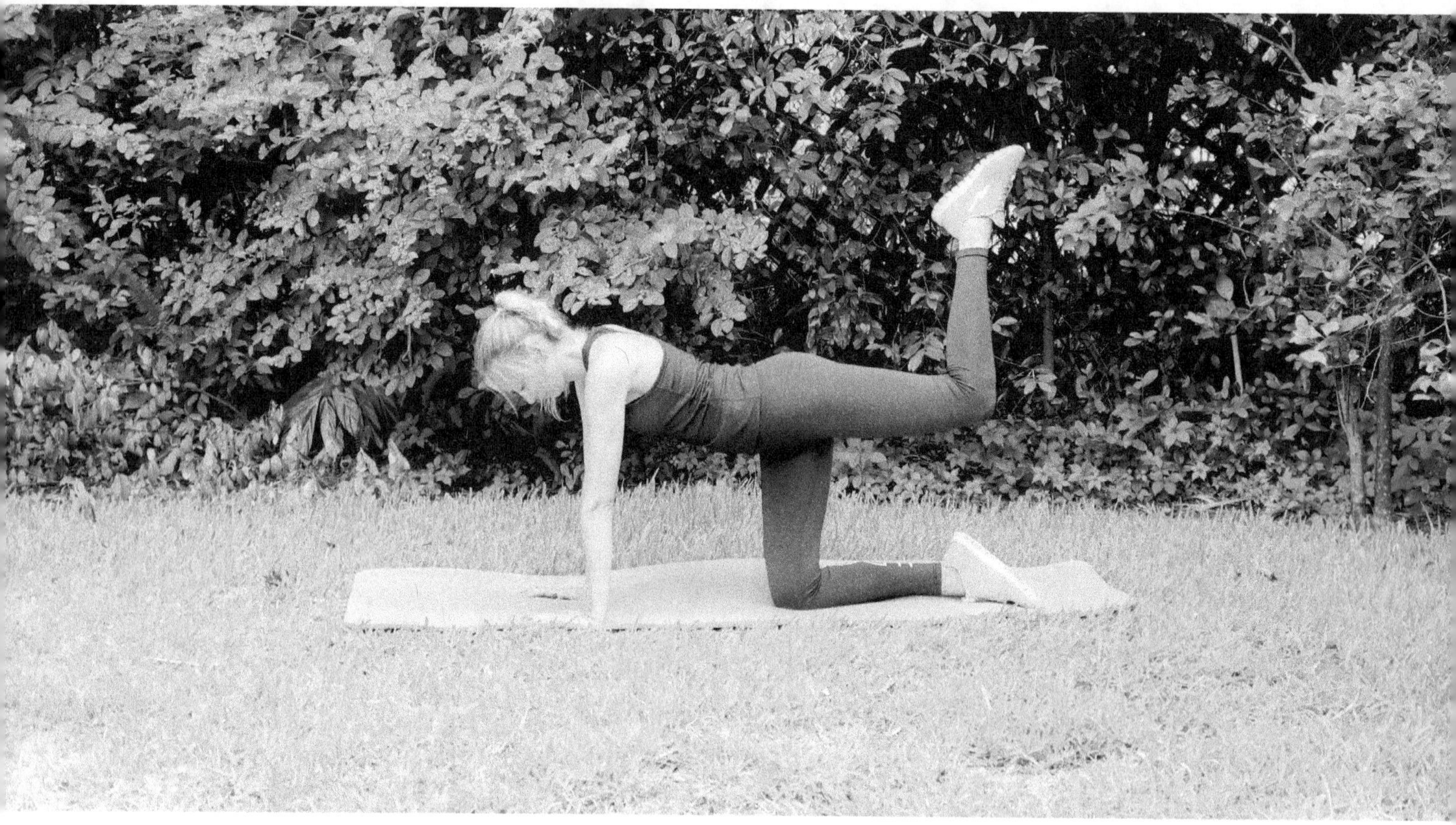

1. *Kneel down on all fours with your legs bent at 90 degrees.*

2. *Bend one knee in and then swing it back to lift it up behind you.*

3. *Return to the starting position and repeat with the opposite leg.*

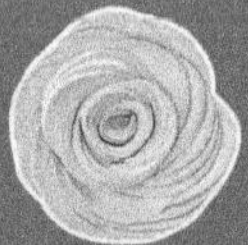

How to do Single-Leg Romanian Deadlifts

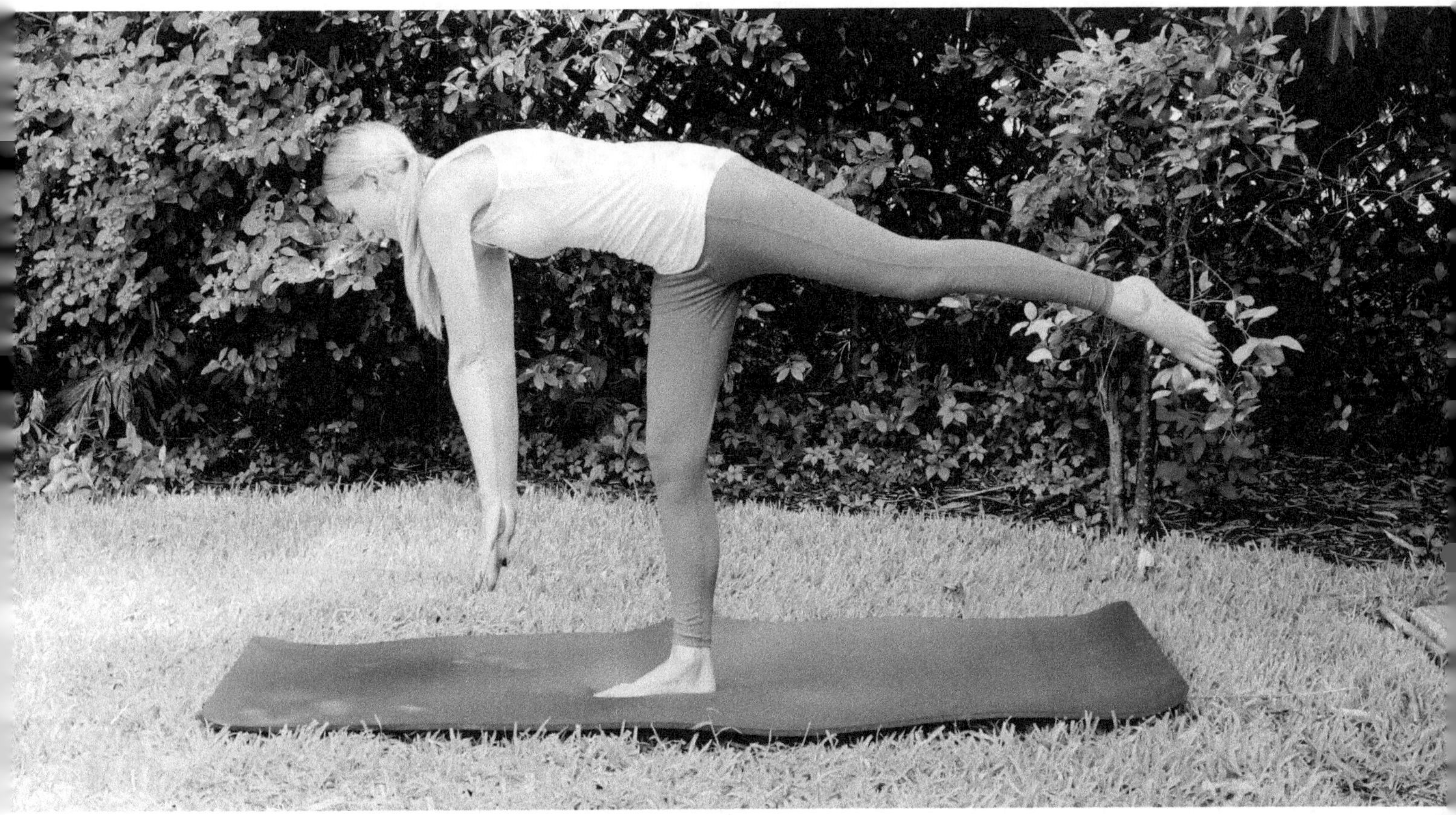

1. Stand with your feet together.

2. Lower your arms and torso in front of you while raising one leg behind your body.

3. Keep the opposite knee slightly bent and reach the arms as close to the floor as possible.

4. To return to the starting position, raise your torso while lowering the back leg and repeat.

5. Then repeat on opposite side.

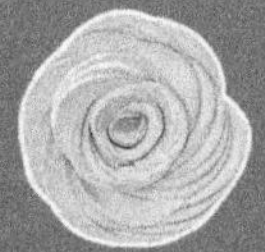

How to do Single-Leg Glute Bridges

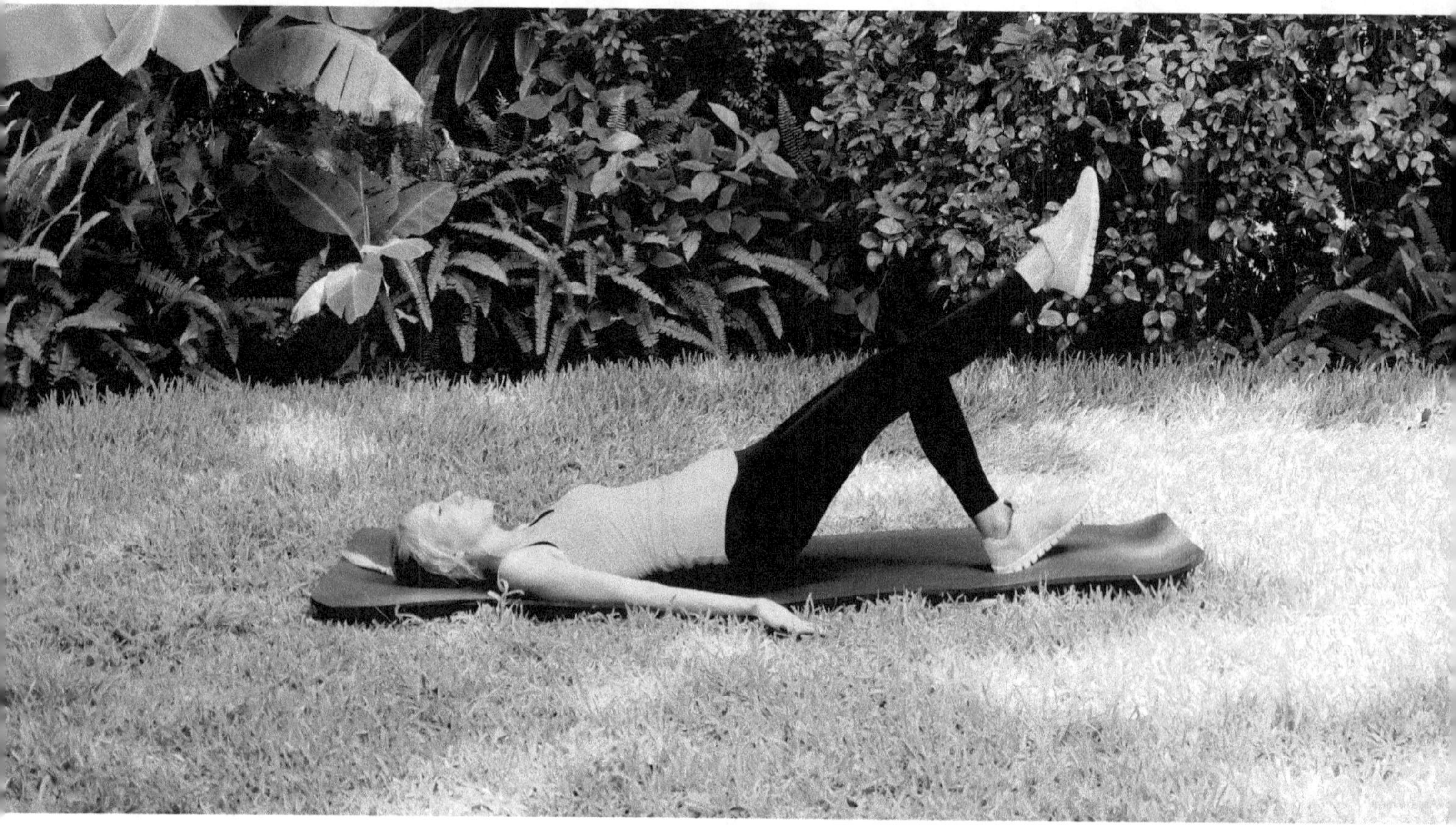

1. Lie on the floor with your hands at your side.

2. Bend one leg and keep one straight.

3. Perform the bridging movement by pushing through your heel on the floor and, squeezing your glutes while lifting your hips off the floor.

4. Hold your position and come down to the start and repeat.

5. Then repeat on opposite side.

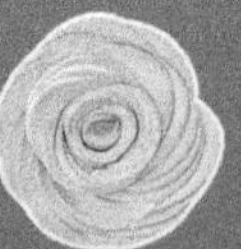

How to do Sit-Ups

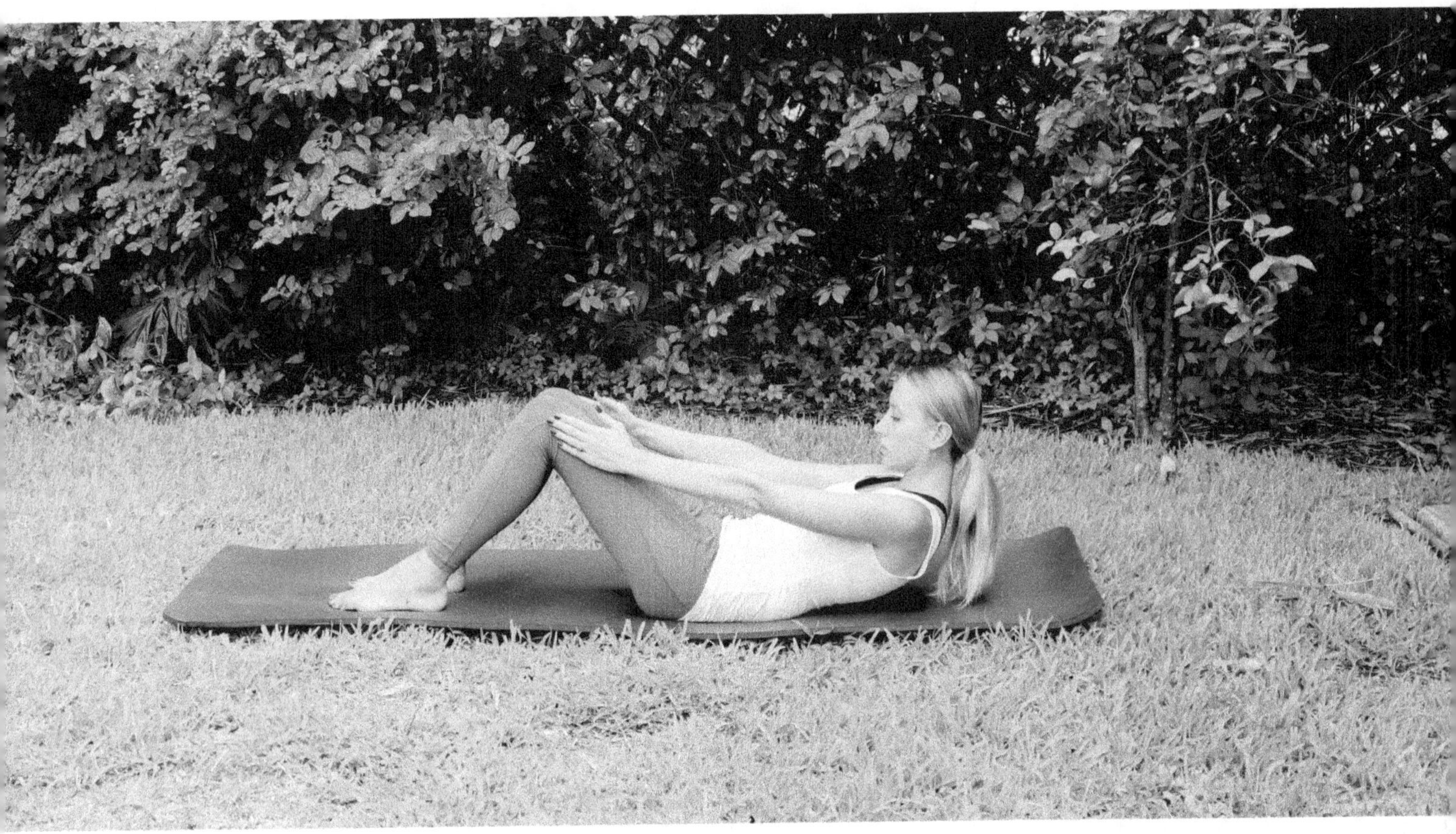

1. *Lying on the ground with your knees bent and your arms at your sides.*

2. *Contract your abs to lift your torso as high as you can off the ground towards your knees, having limited movement in the lower back.*

3. *Repeat.*

How to do Twisting Sit-Ups

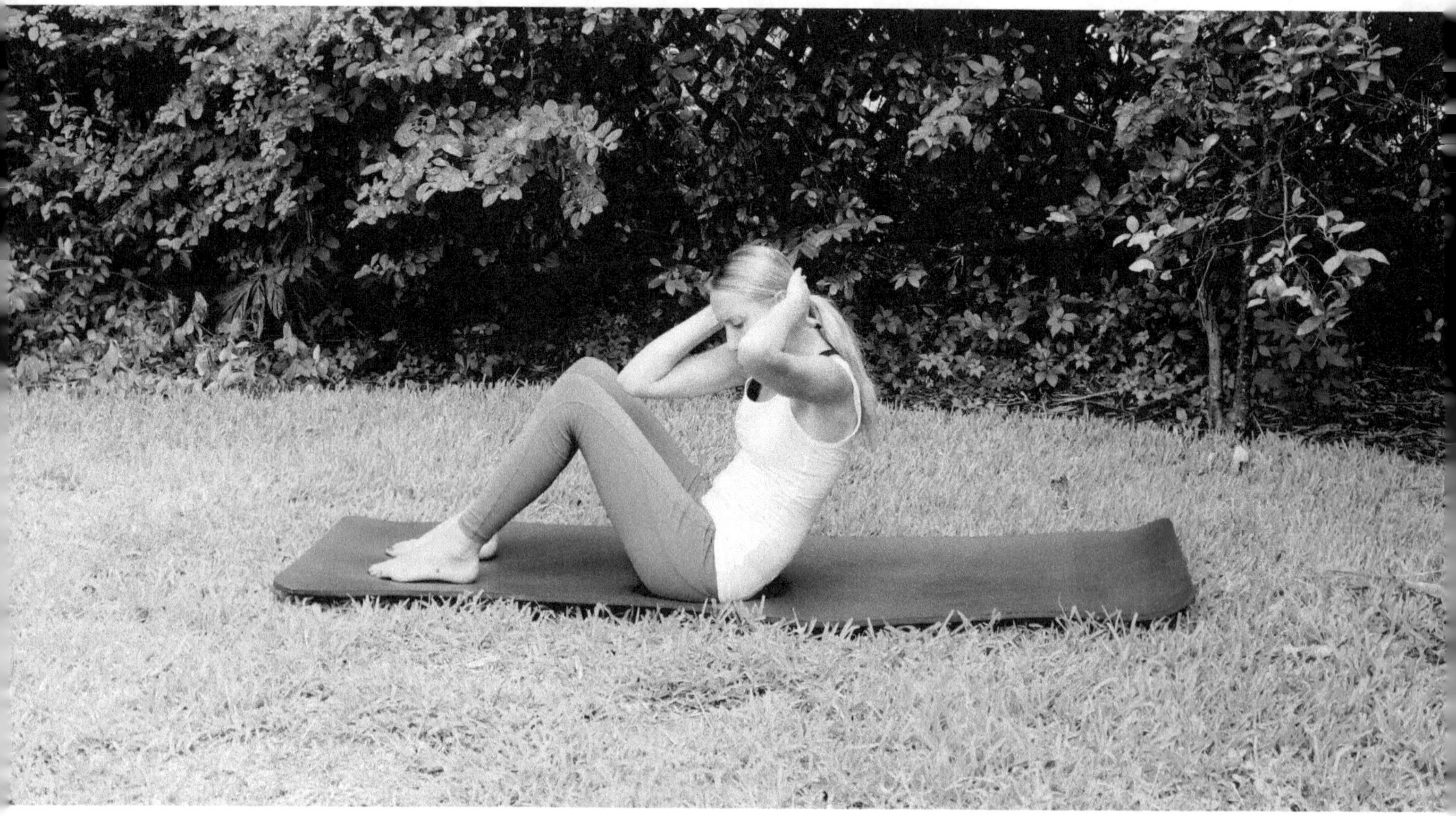

1. *Lying on the ground with your knees bent and hands behind your head.*

2. *Contract your abs to lift your torso as high as you can off the ground towards your knees.*

3. *At the top of the movement bring your opposite elbow towards your opposite knee, having limited movement in the lower back.*

4. *Repeat.*

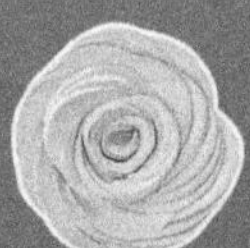

How to do Crunches

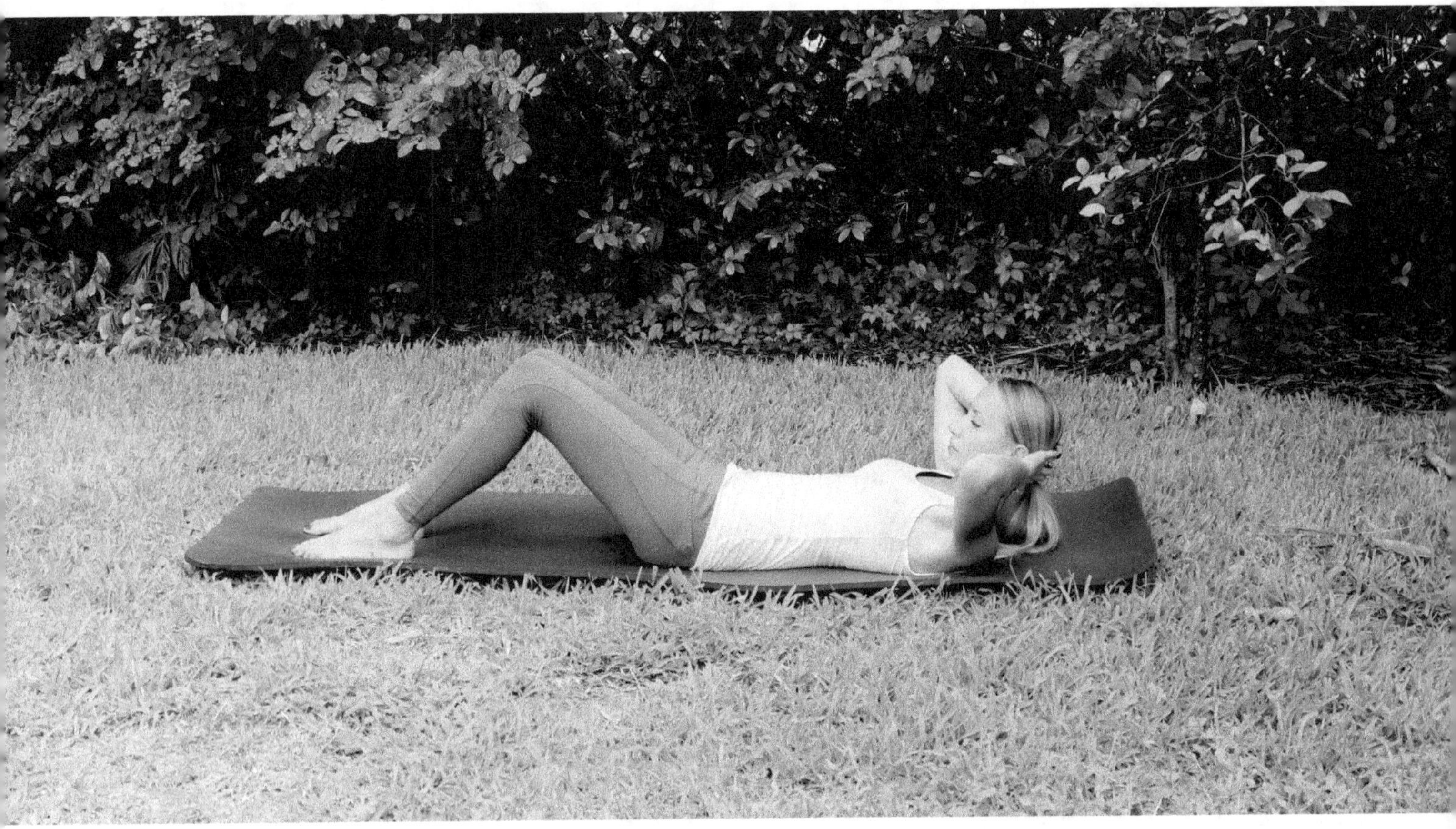

1. *Lie on your back with your knees bent and feet flat on the floor.*

2. *With your hands behind your head, contract your core and curl your upper back up from the floor.*

3. *Hold briefly, and then lower yourself back down.*

4. *Repeat.*

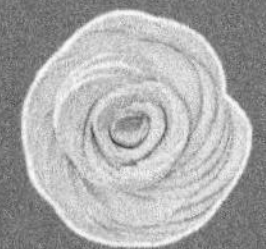

How to do Side Crunches

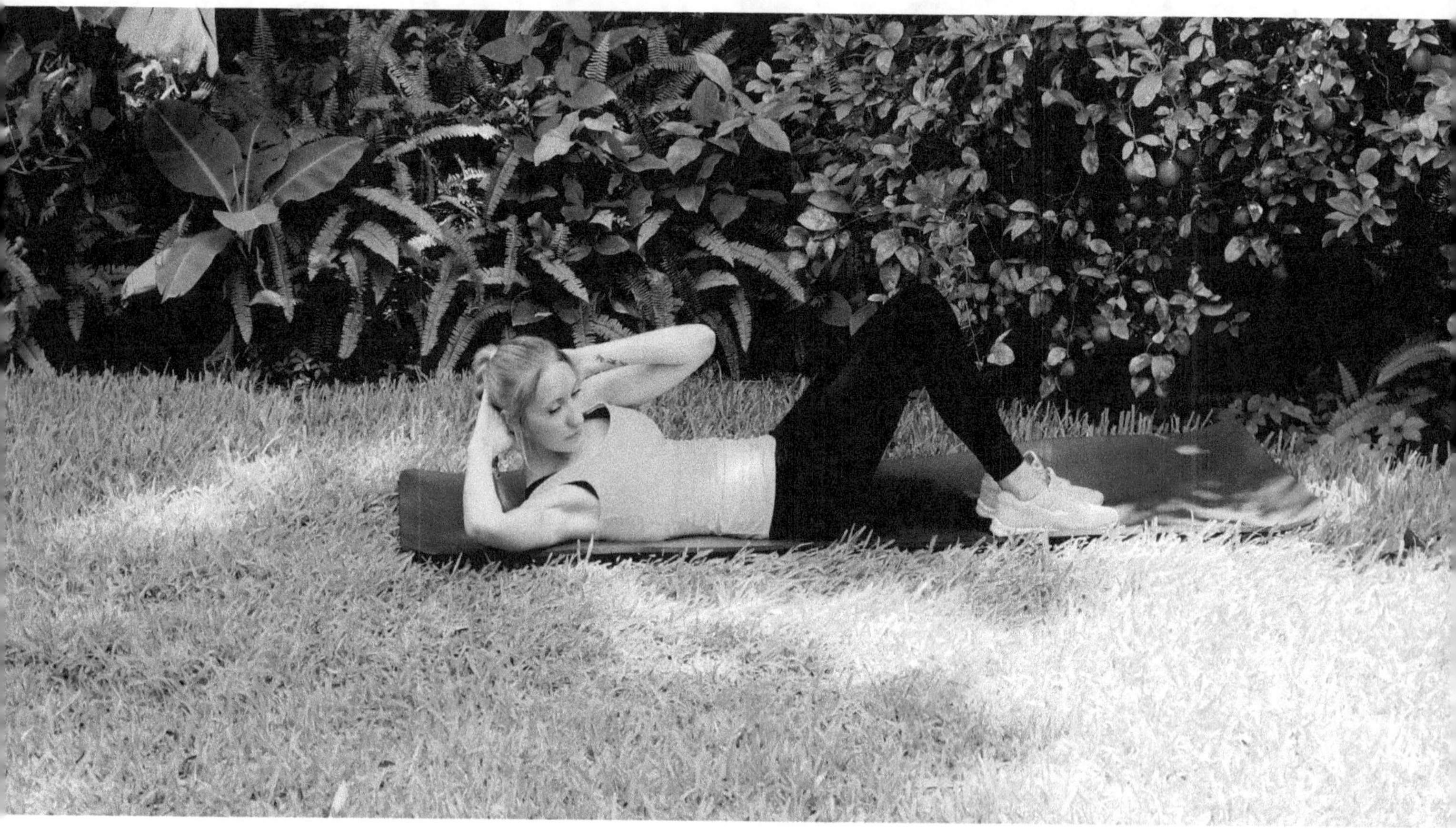

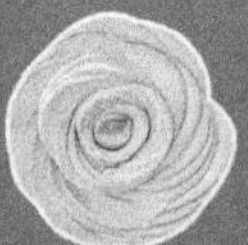

1. Set up in the same position as the regular crunch.

2. As you lift your upper body up from the floor, keep your hands behind your head and reach one of your elbows towards the opposite knee.

3. Repeat.

How to do Flutter Kicks

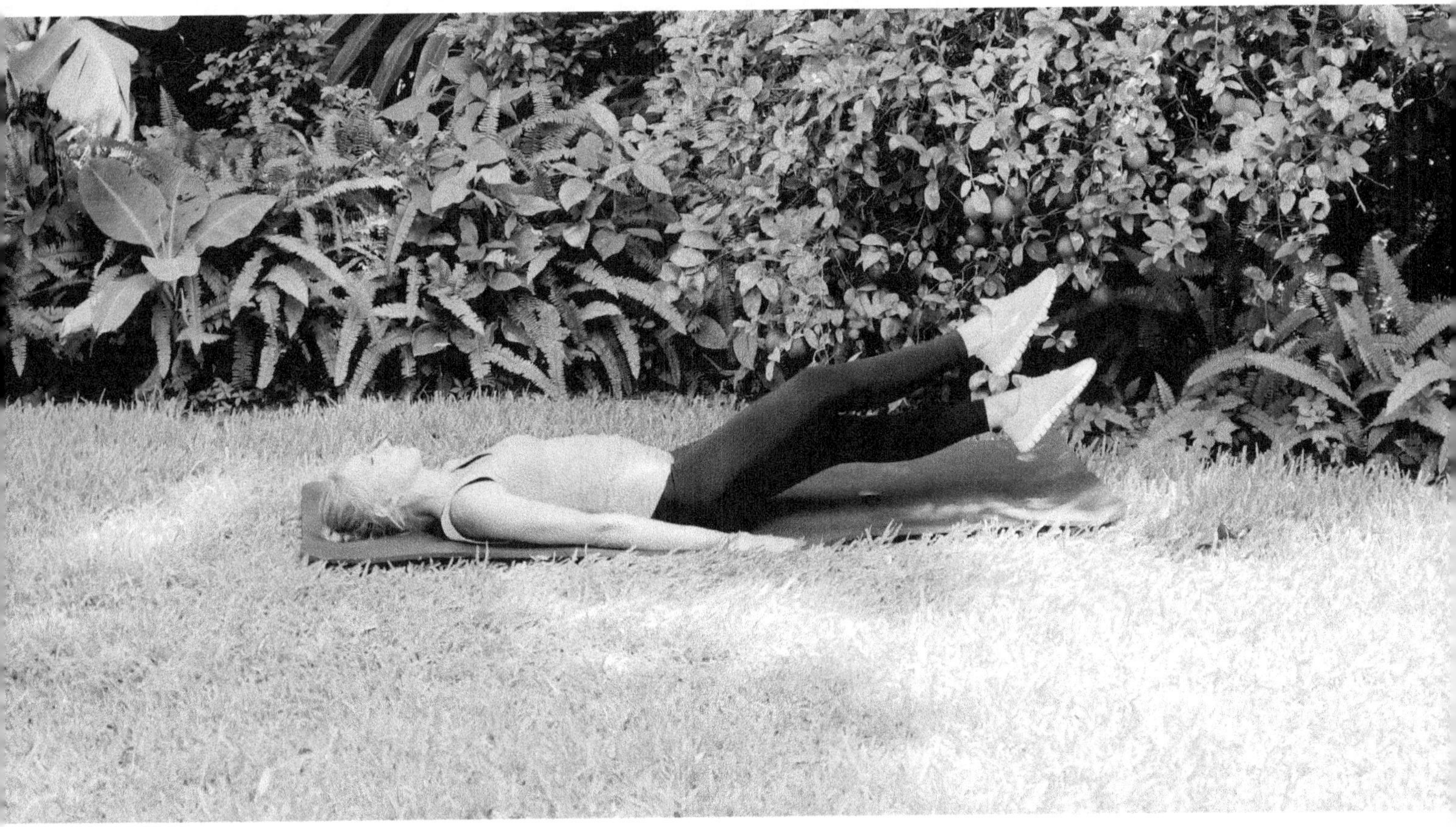

1. *Lie on your back with arms at your sides and palms facing down.*

2. *With your legs extended, lift your heels a few inches off the ground.*

3. *Engage your core, and make small up-and-down kicks with your legs.*

How to do Bicycles

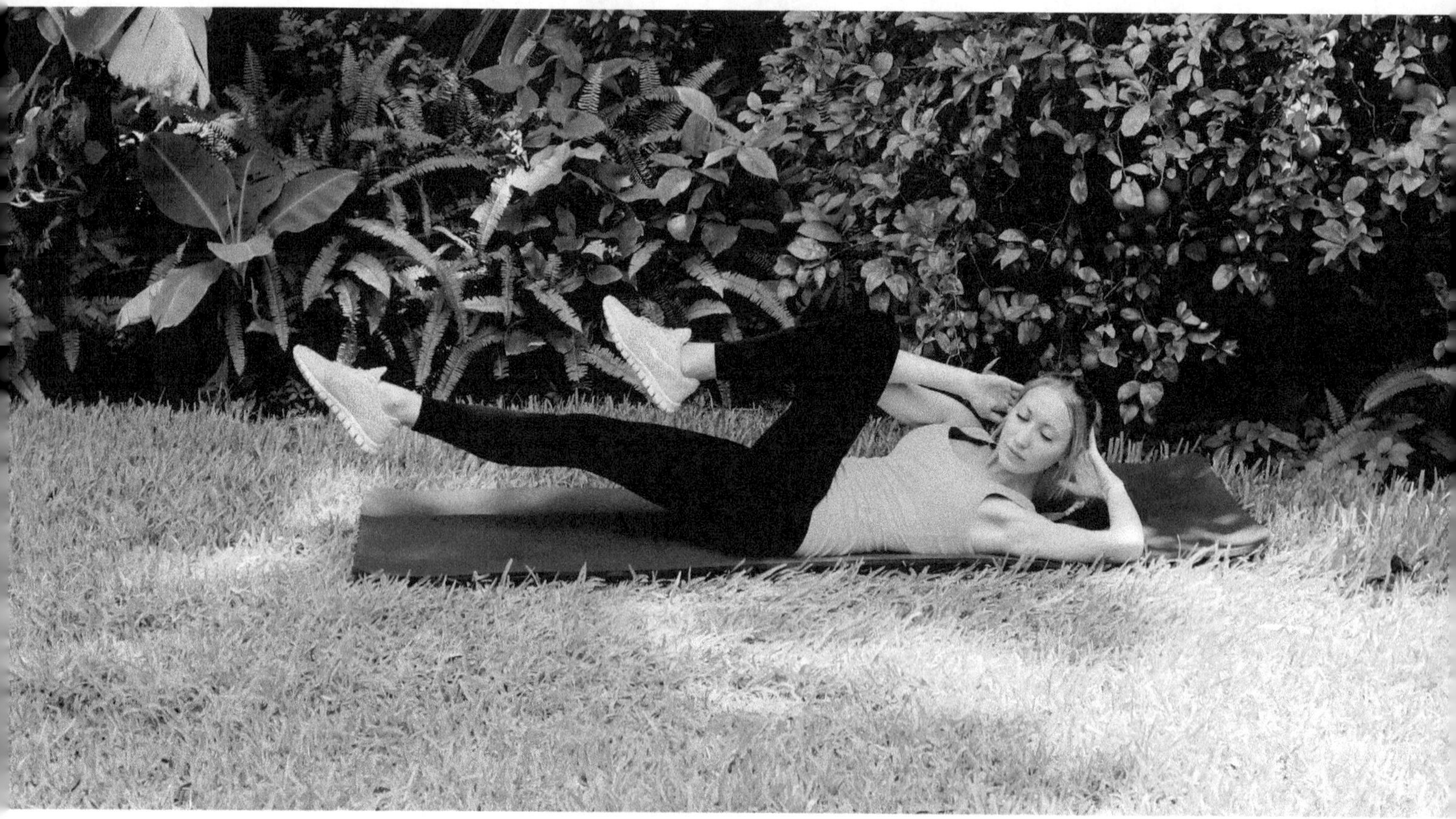

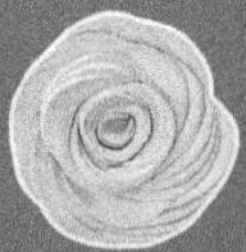

1. Lie down on the ground with your knees bent and hands behind your head.

2. Lift your legs off the ground and make a pedalling motion, like you are riding a bicycle.

3. With your hands behind your head, bring your opposing elbow to meet each leg as it comes toward you.

How to do Supermans

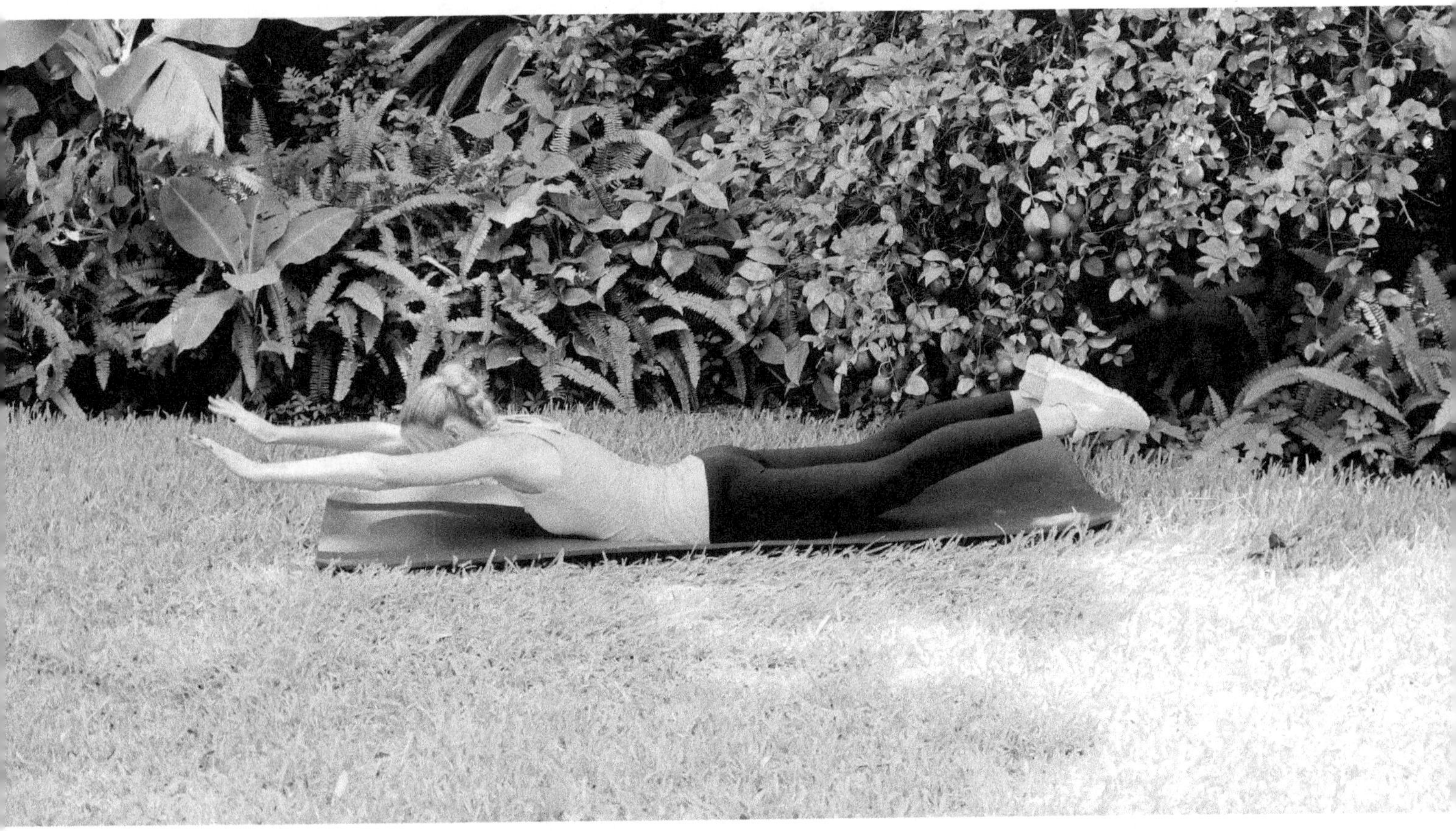

1. *Lie face-down on the ground with your arms outstretched in front of you.*

2. *Simultaneously lift your arms, legs and torso off the ground and focus on squeezing your glutes throughout.*

How to do Bird Dogs

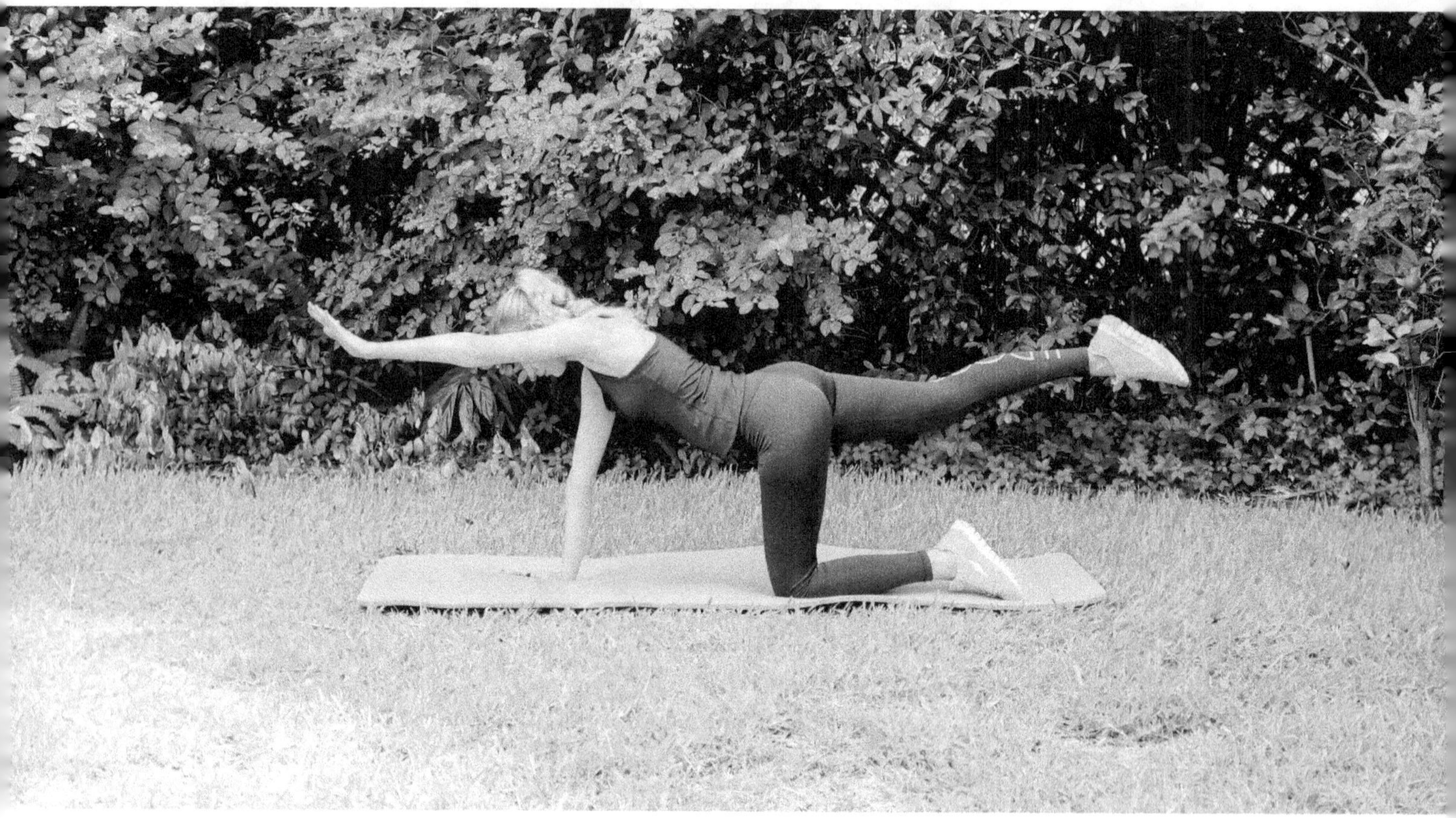

1. Start on all fours with your back flat.

2. Raise one arm forward while simultaneously lifting your opposite leg until both limbs are in line with your torso.

3. Slowly bring your leg and arm back to the starting position and then repeat with the opposite limbs.

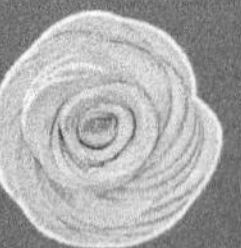

How to do Dead Bugs

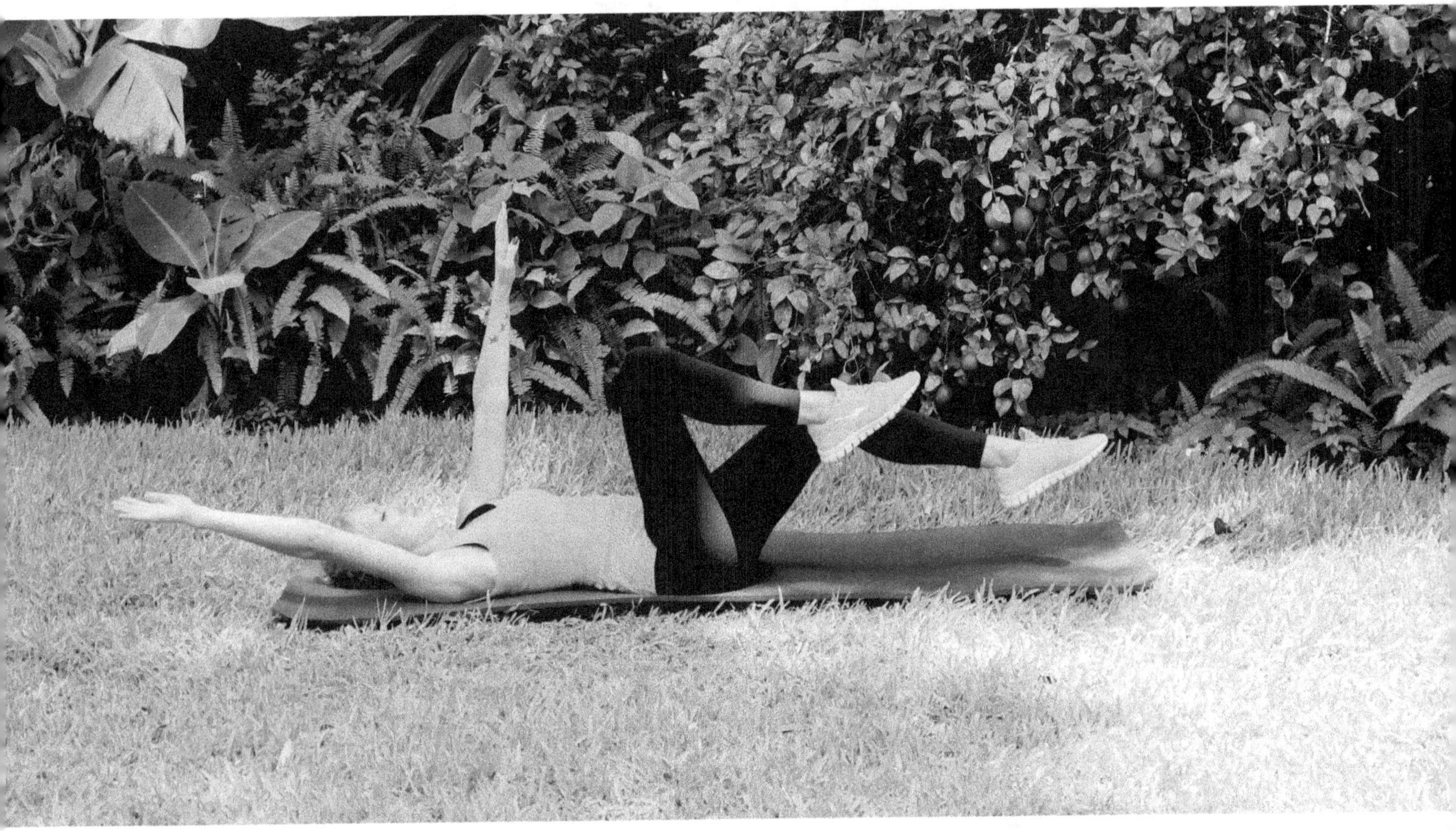

1. Lie flat on your back with your knees bent at 90 degrees and your arms
   pointing upwards.

2. Flatten your back against the floor and exhale as you lower one leg and
   your opposing arm until they are just hovering above the ground.

3. Pause, return to the starting position, and then repeat with your opposing
   limbs.

How to do Planks

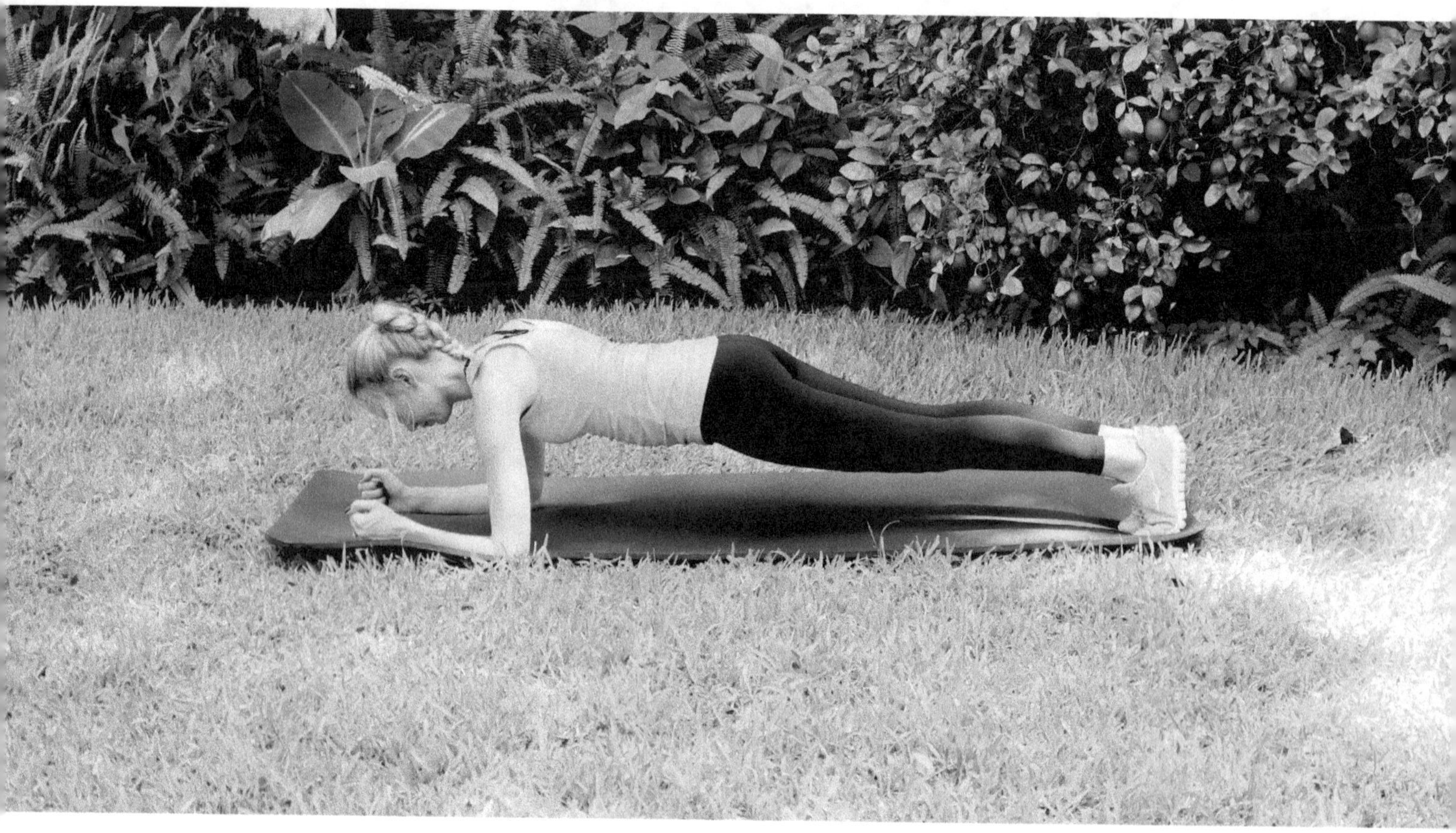

1. Lie face down with your forearms on the floor and fist your hands.

2. Extend the legs behind you and rise up onto your toes.

3. Keeping the back straight, tighten your core, quads and glutes and hold the position for as long as you can.

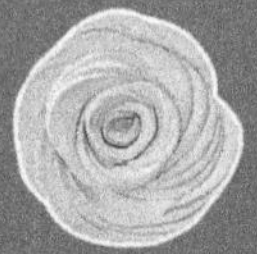

How to do Feet-Elevated Planks

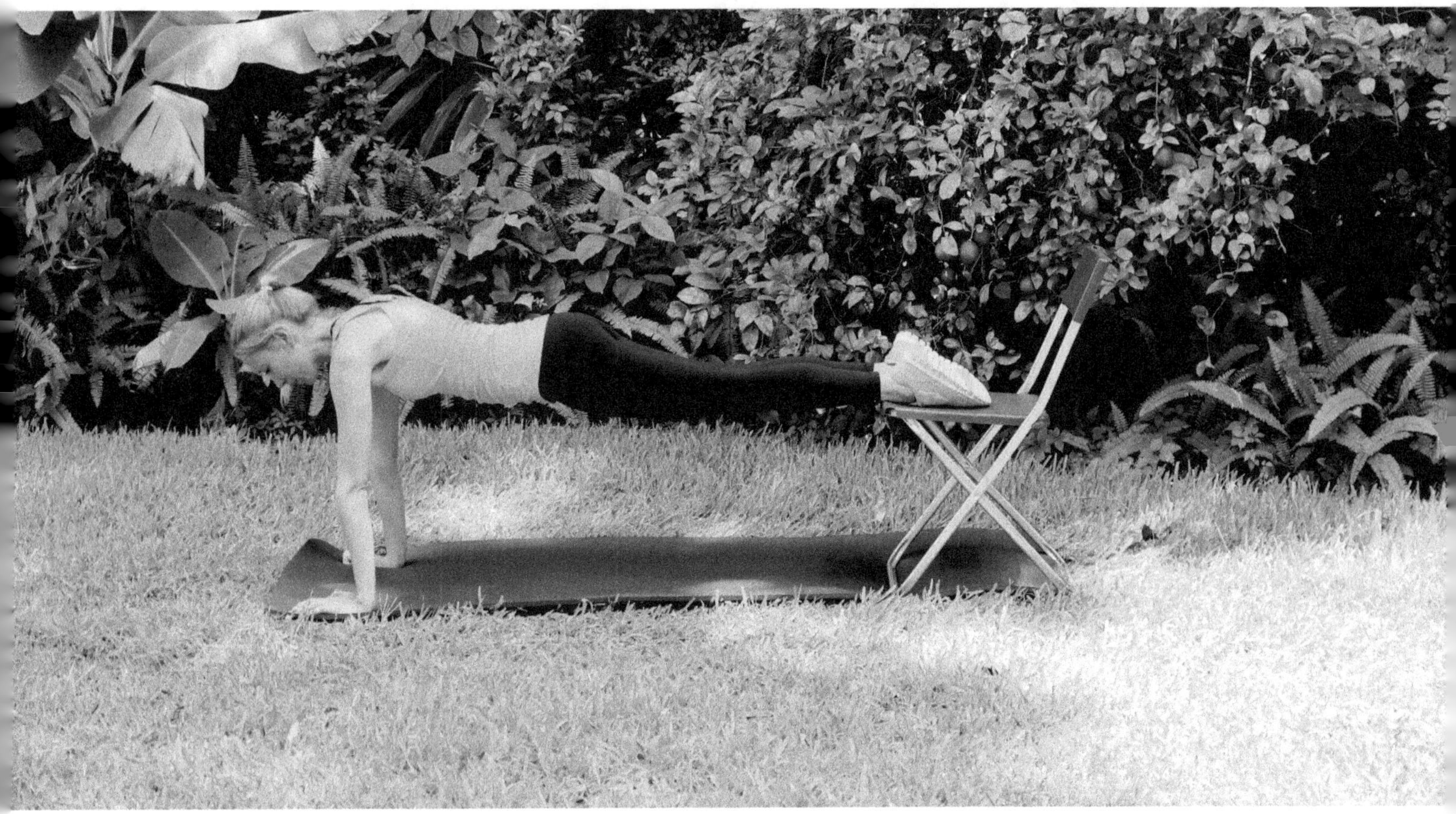

1. To make the conventional plank more difficult, find a raised surface such as a chair or low table.

2. Extend your legs behind you with your feet downwards on the raised surface.

3. Holding your upper body with your arms straight and palms on the floor.

4. Hold the position for as long as you can.

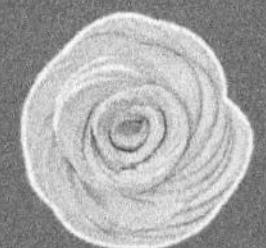

How to do Side Planks

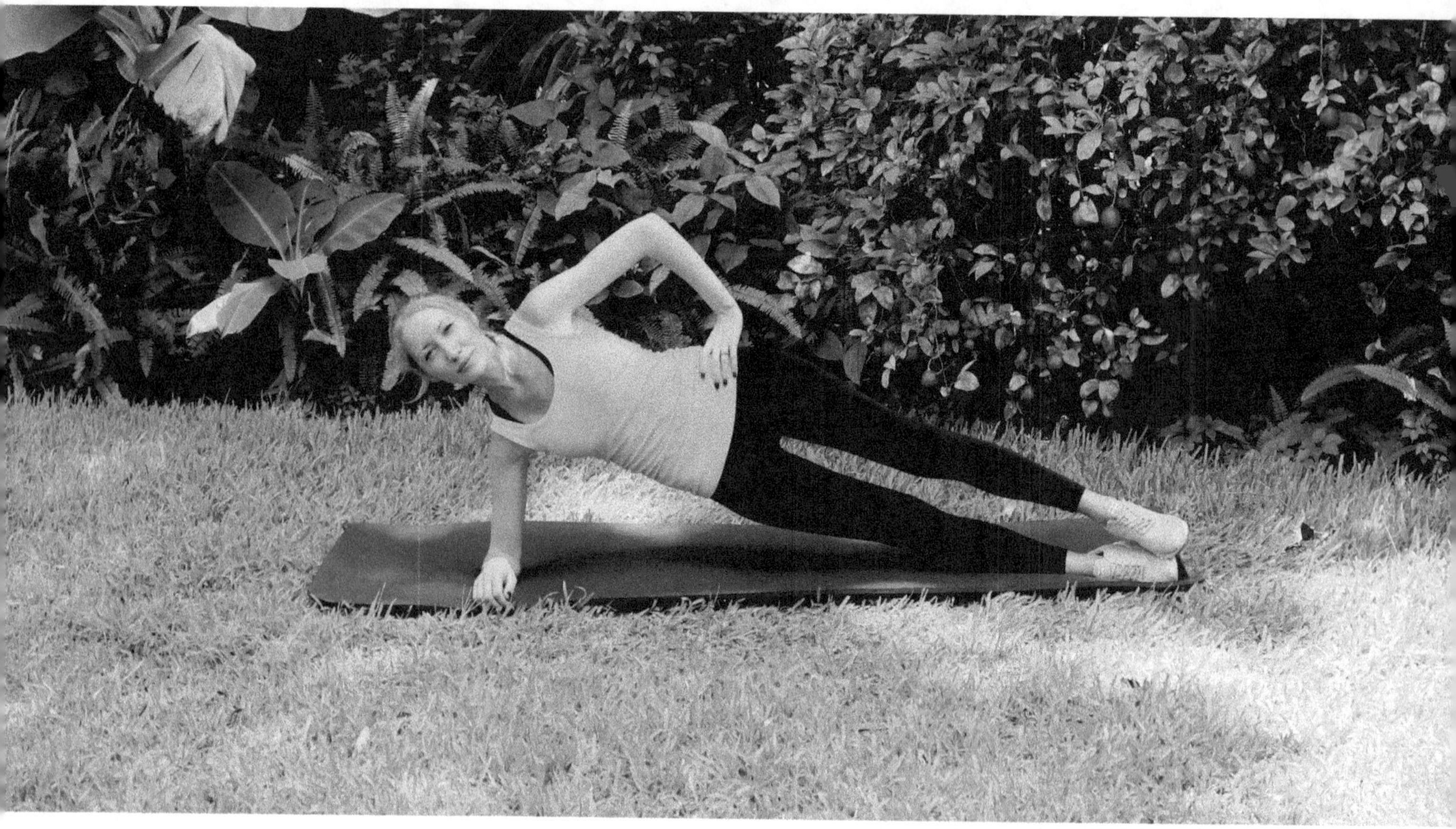

1. Lay on your side, with just one foot and one forearm touching the ground.

2. Raise your body up and keep your body in a straight line.

3. Hold the position for as long as you can.

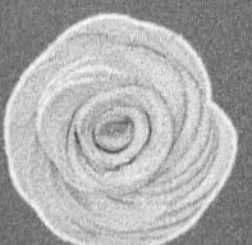

How to do Lying Straight-Leg Raises

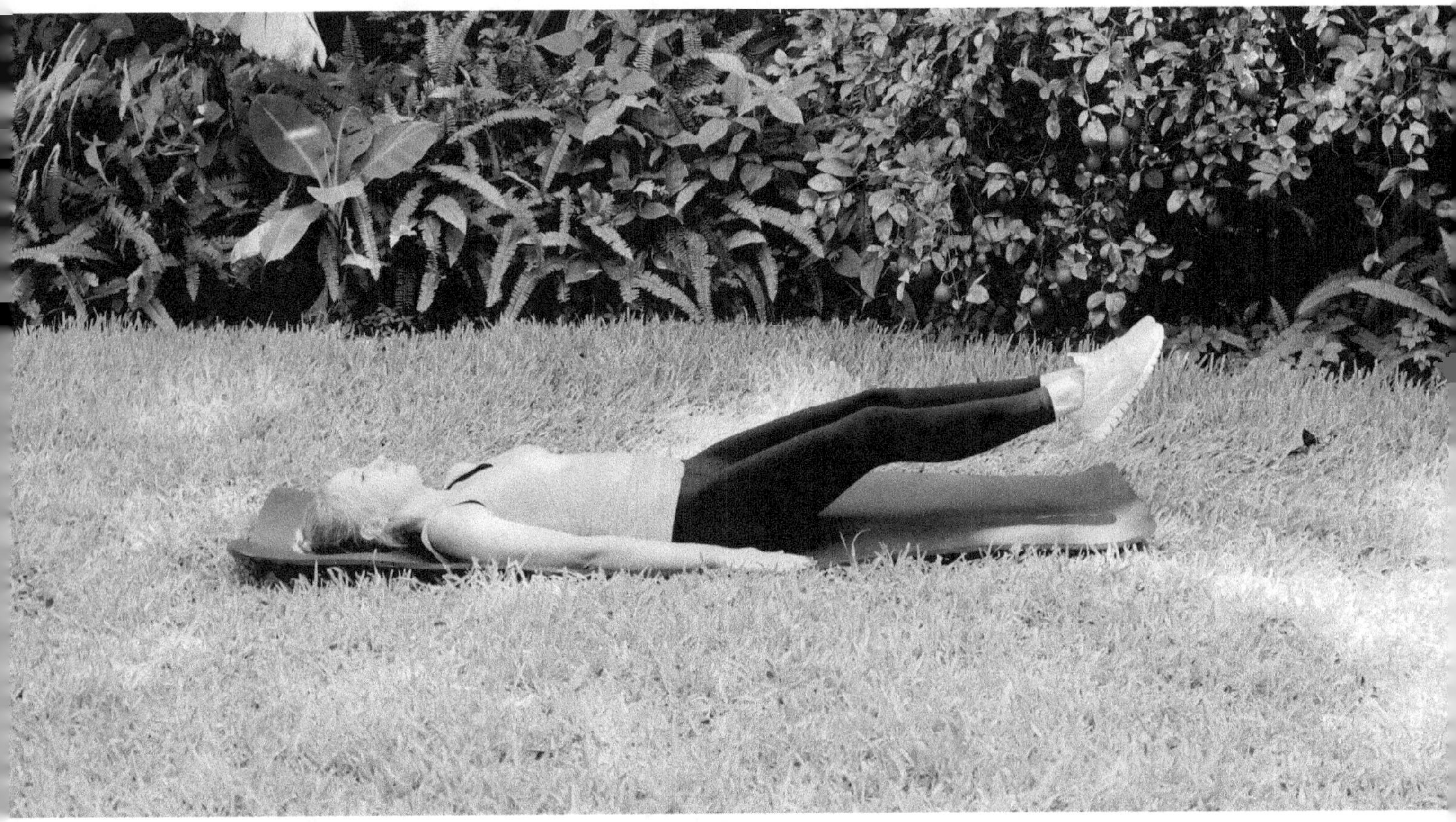

1. Lie flat on the ground with your legs straight.

2. Contract your abdominals and lift your legs until your hips are bent at 90 degrees.

3. Lower the legs slowly to the ground and repeat.

How to do Bent Knees Windshield Wipers

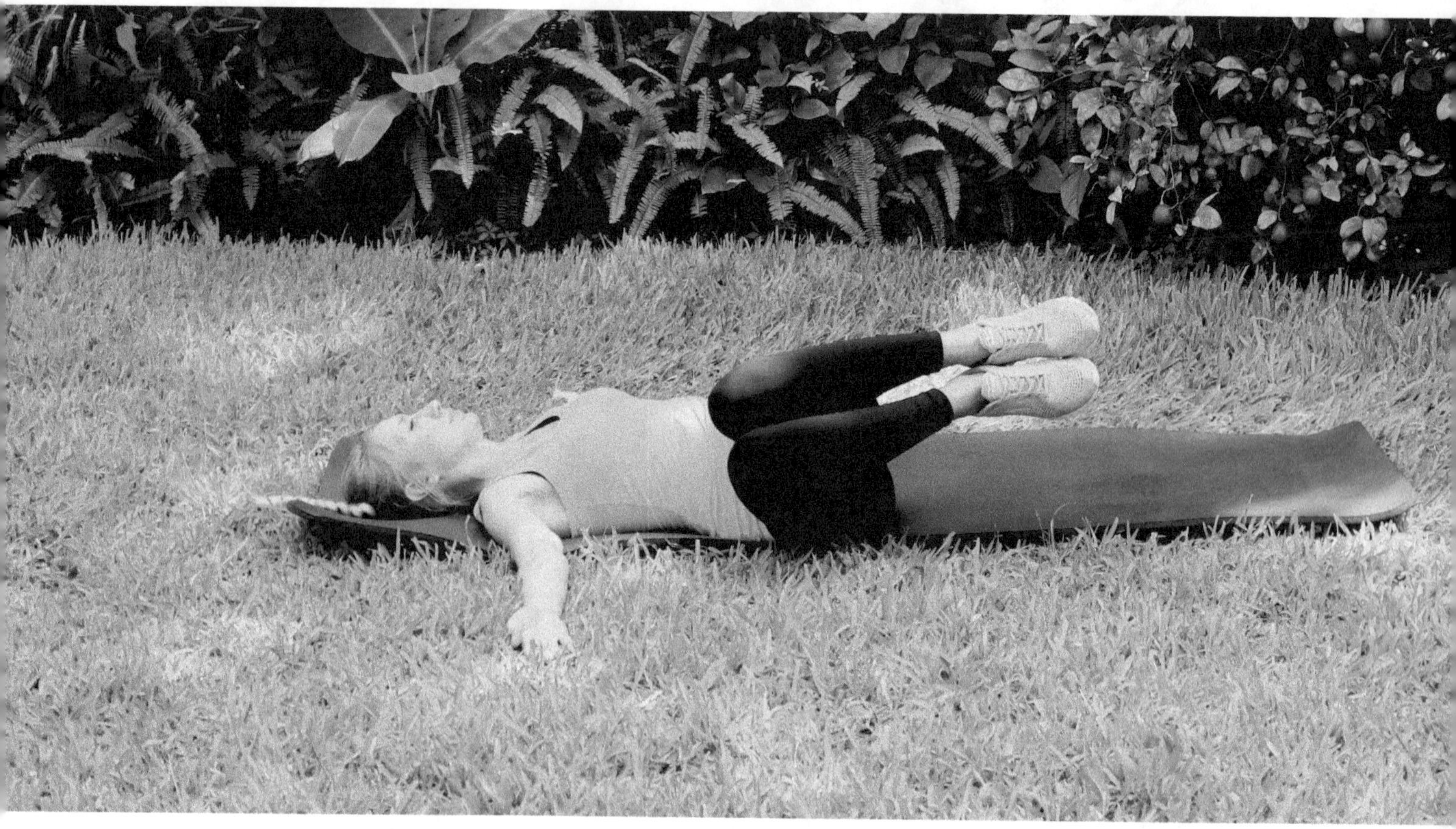

1. Lying on your back with your arms spread wide for stability, lift your legs and bend your knees.

2. Keeping your core tight, rotate your bent legs slowly from side to side.

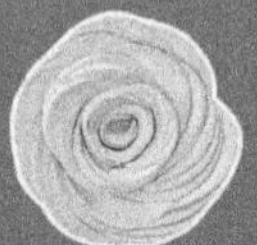

How to do Push-Ups

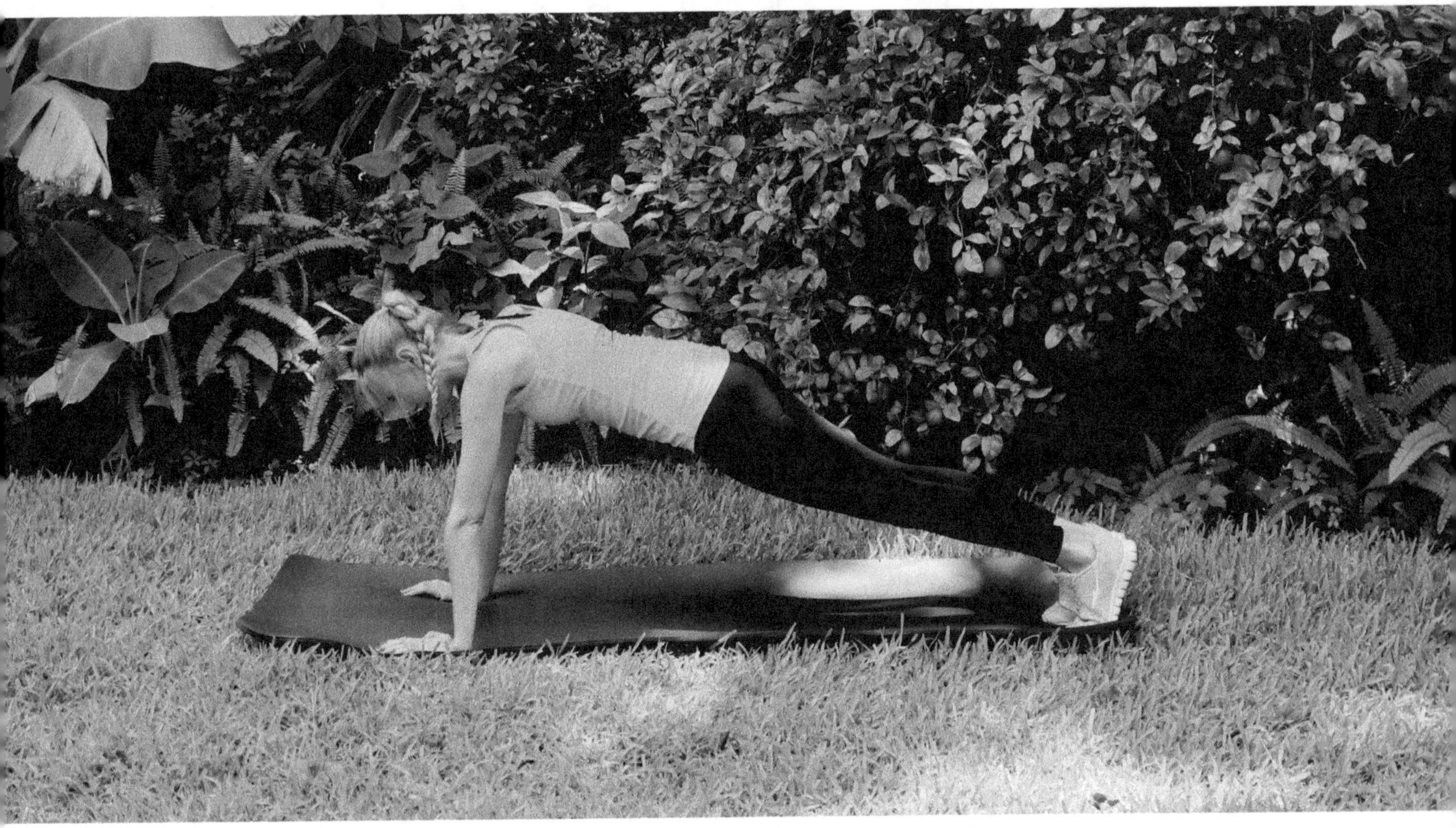

1. *Position your hands shoulder-width apart and brace your core to make your body into a straight line. You can either be on your toes or bend your knees for more support.*

2. *Bend at the elbows until your chest touches the floor, and then quickly push back up to return to the starting position.*

3. *Keep your elbows close to your body throughout and repeat.*

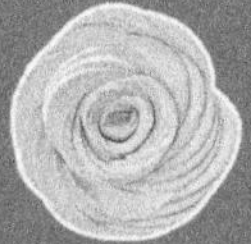

How to do Crab Walks

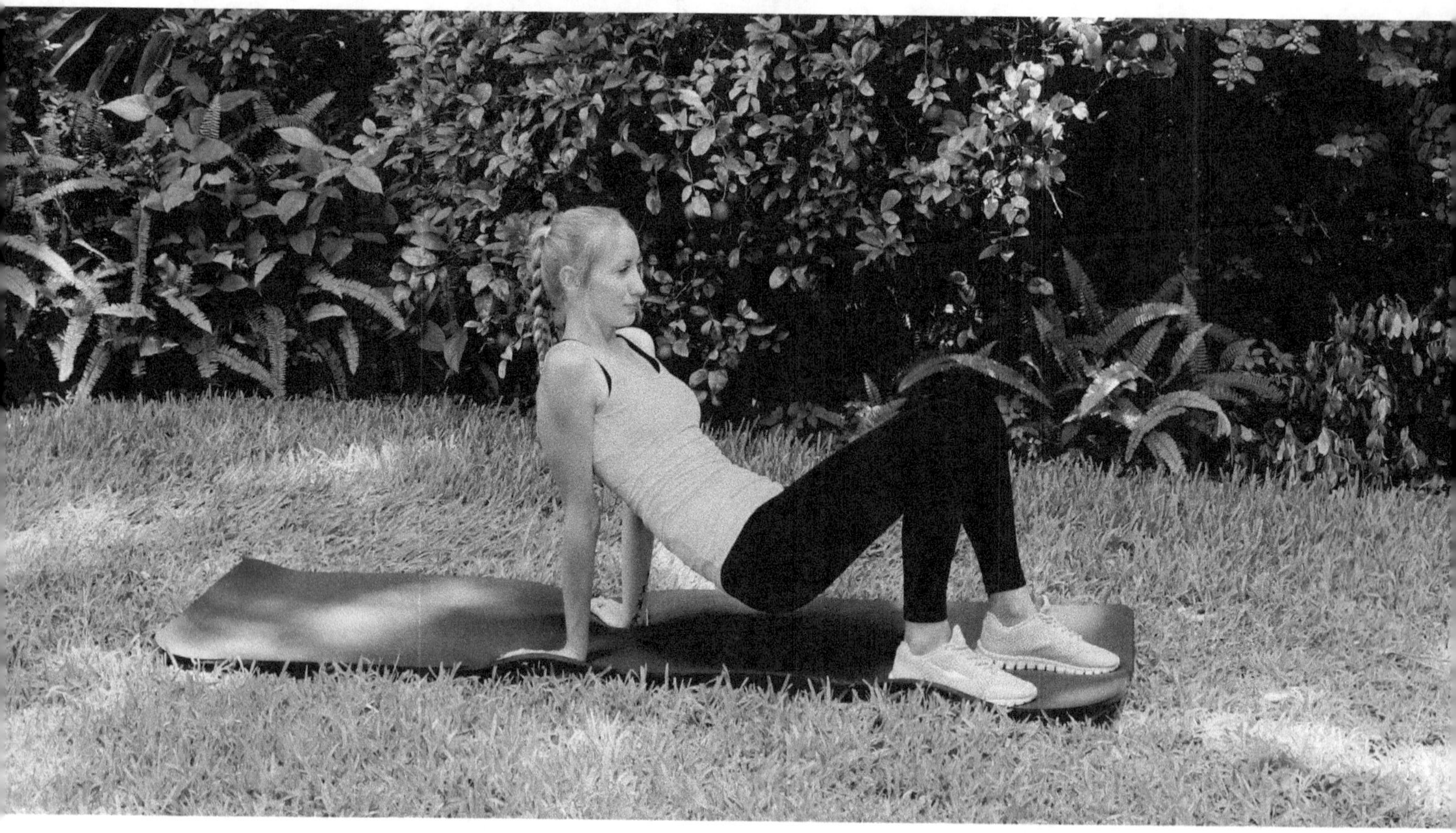

1. Facing up, use your hands and feet to lift your body off the ground.

2. Keeping your hips high, walk yourself backwards using same-side patterns of leg and arm movement.

3. After going backwards, reverse the movement to go forwards and return to the start.

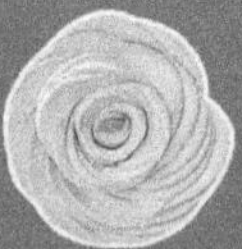

How to do Mountain Climbers

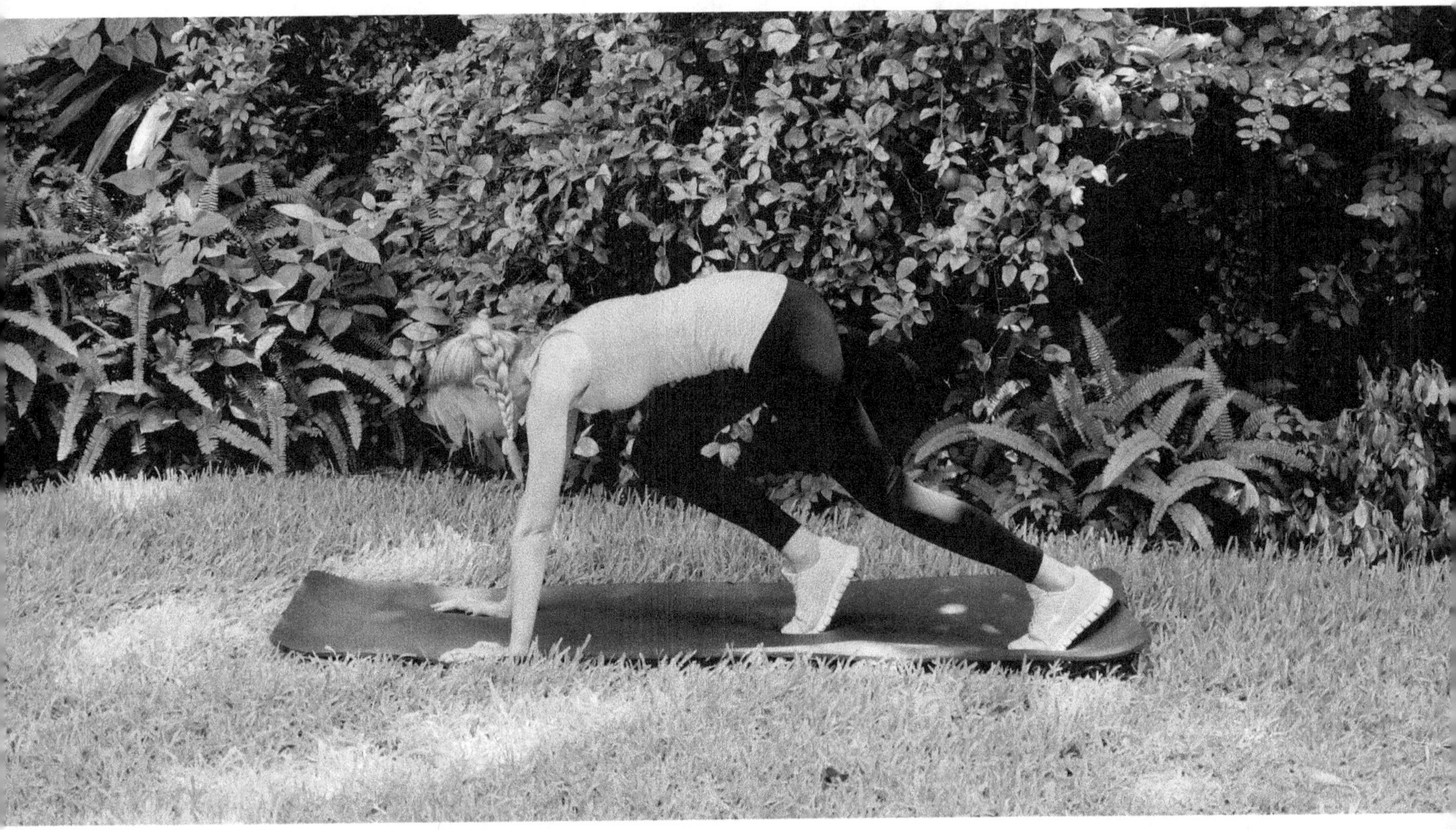

1. *Start on your hands and knees.*

2. *Then bring the left knee forward directly under the chest while straightening the right leg.*

3. *With your hands on the ground and core tight, jump and switch legs. The left leg should now be extended behind the body with the right knee forward.*

4. *Repeat.*

How to do Jumping Jacks

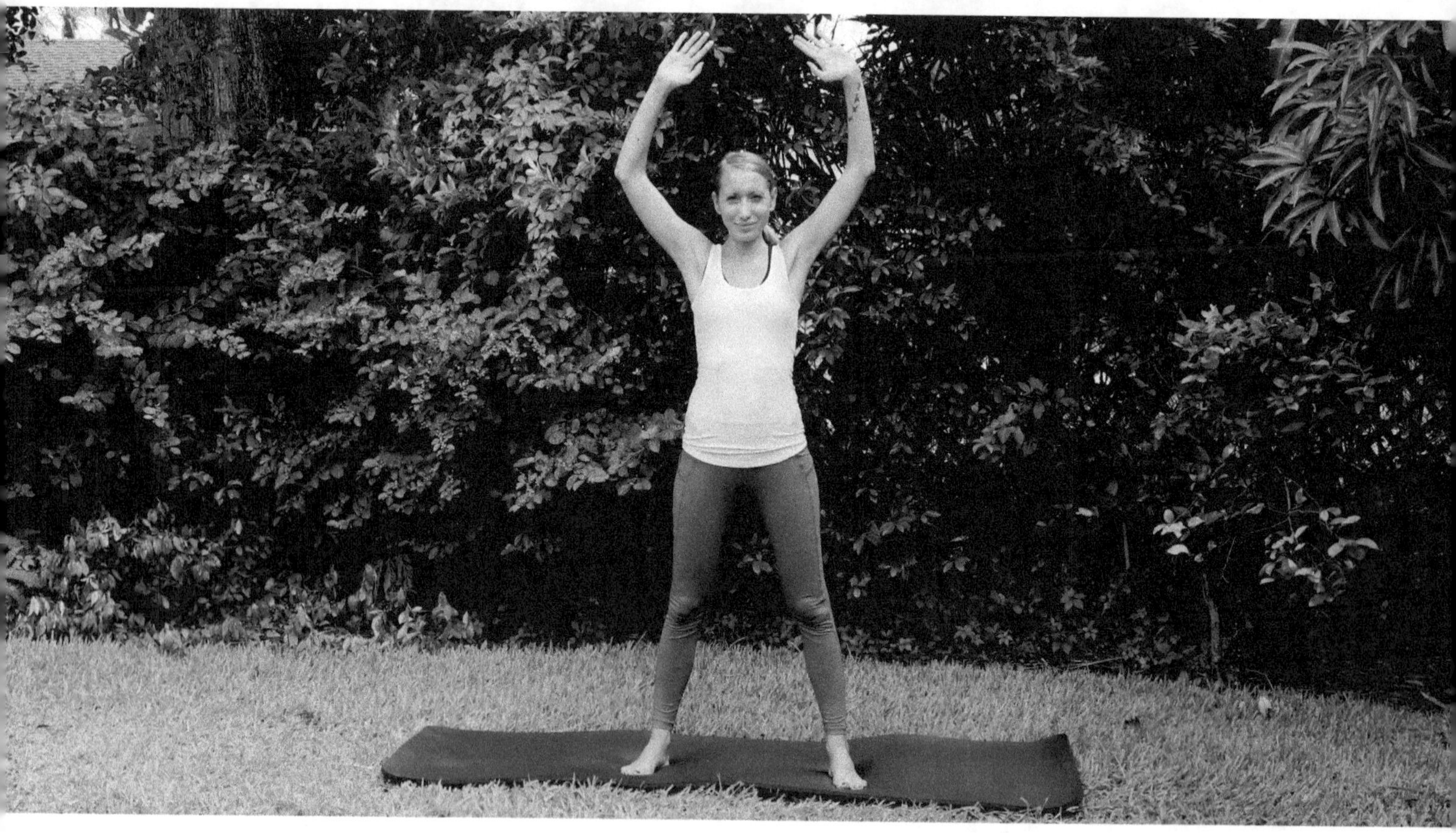

1. In a standing position, jump and spread your legs to your side while simultaneously lifting the arms.

2. As soon as you land spring back into the starting position and repeat.

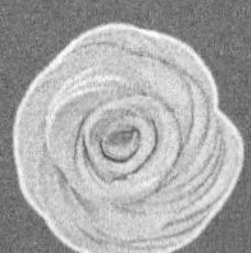

How to do Jumping Rope

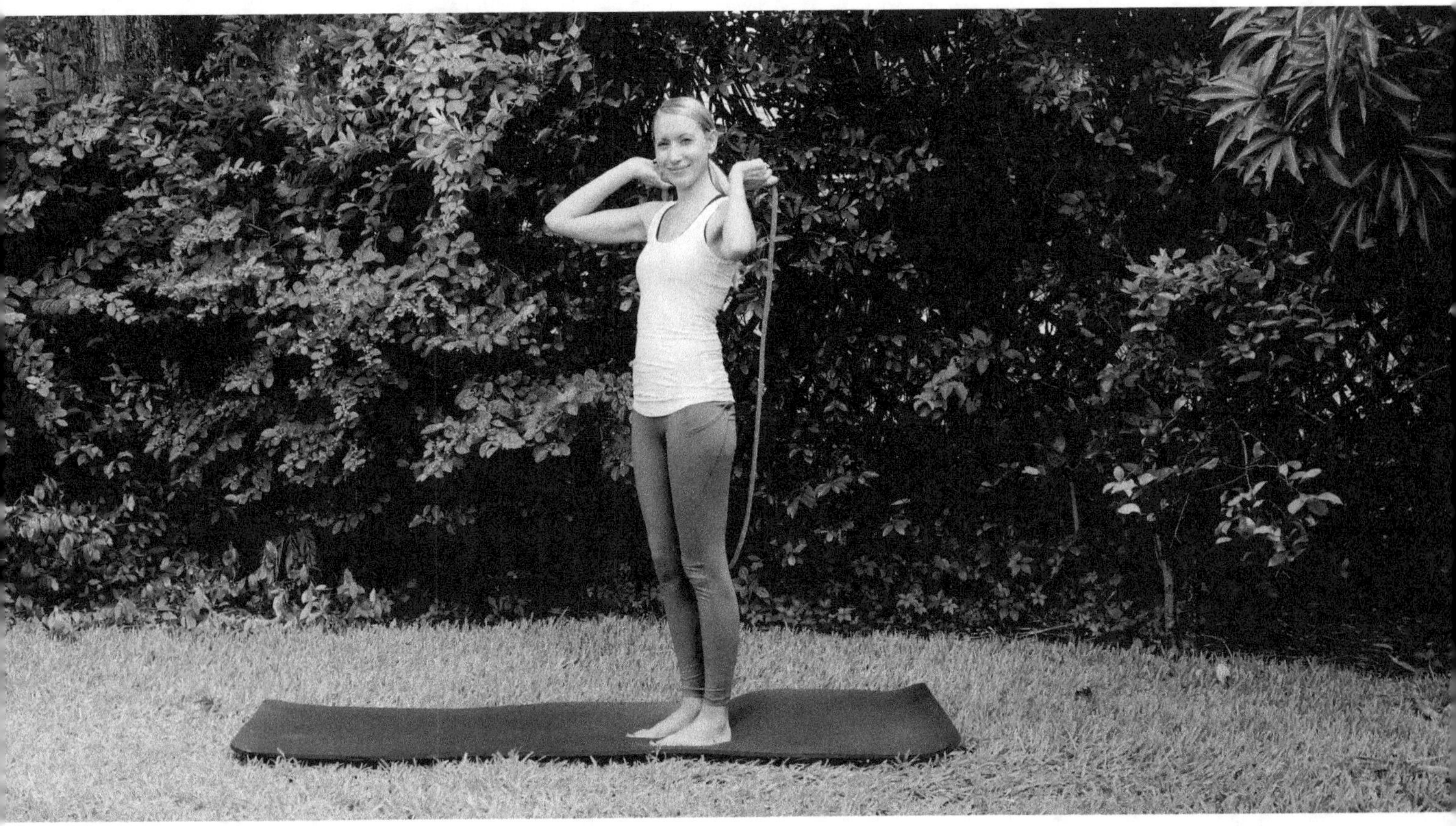

1. With a skipping rope, hold each end, one in each hand with the rope behind you.

2. Swing the rope over the top of your body and when it comes around jump over it with both feet.

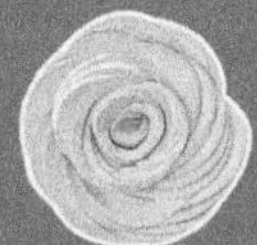

How to do Lateral Jumps

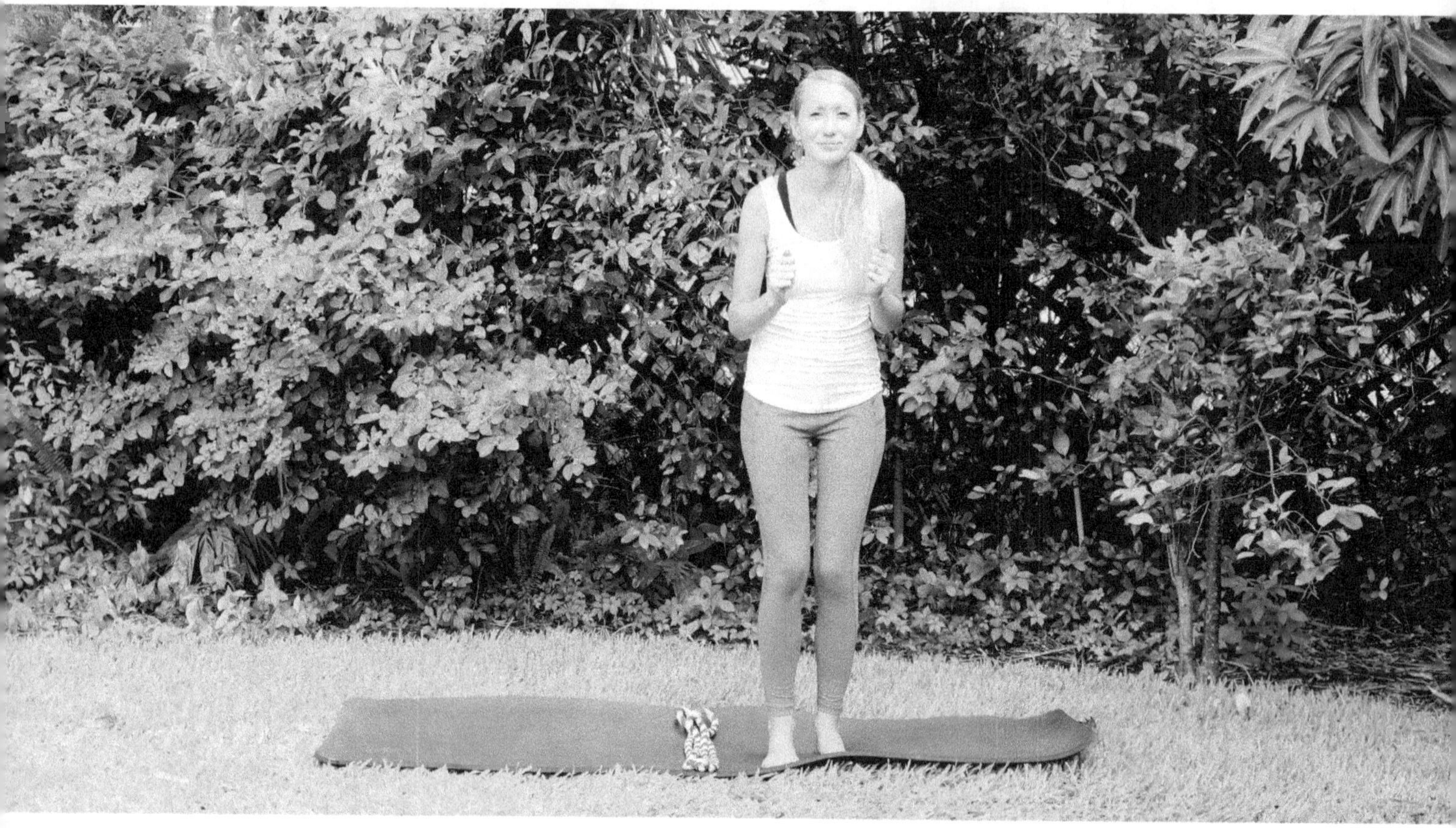

1. In a standing position, jump side-to-side, or find something to jump over instead.

2. Keep your feet together and lift your knees as you jump and land as softly as possible.

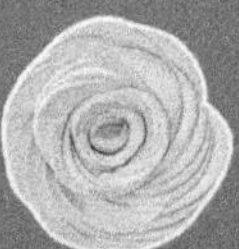

How to do Jumping Lunges

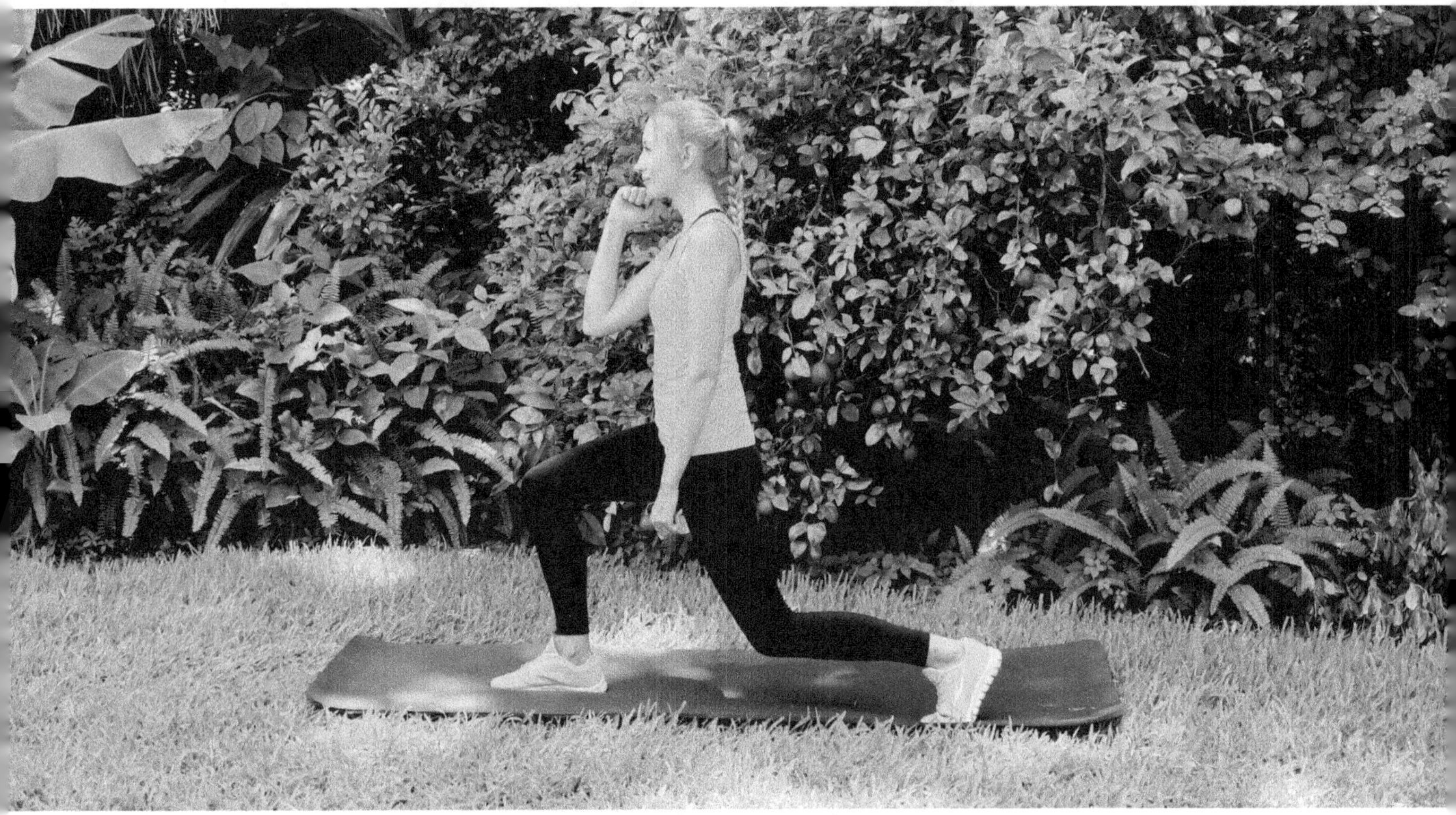

1. Jump into the air and alternate legs each time.

2. Spring straight up into the air as high as possible and absorb the landing by sinking into a lunge position.

3. Repeat.

How to do Burpees

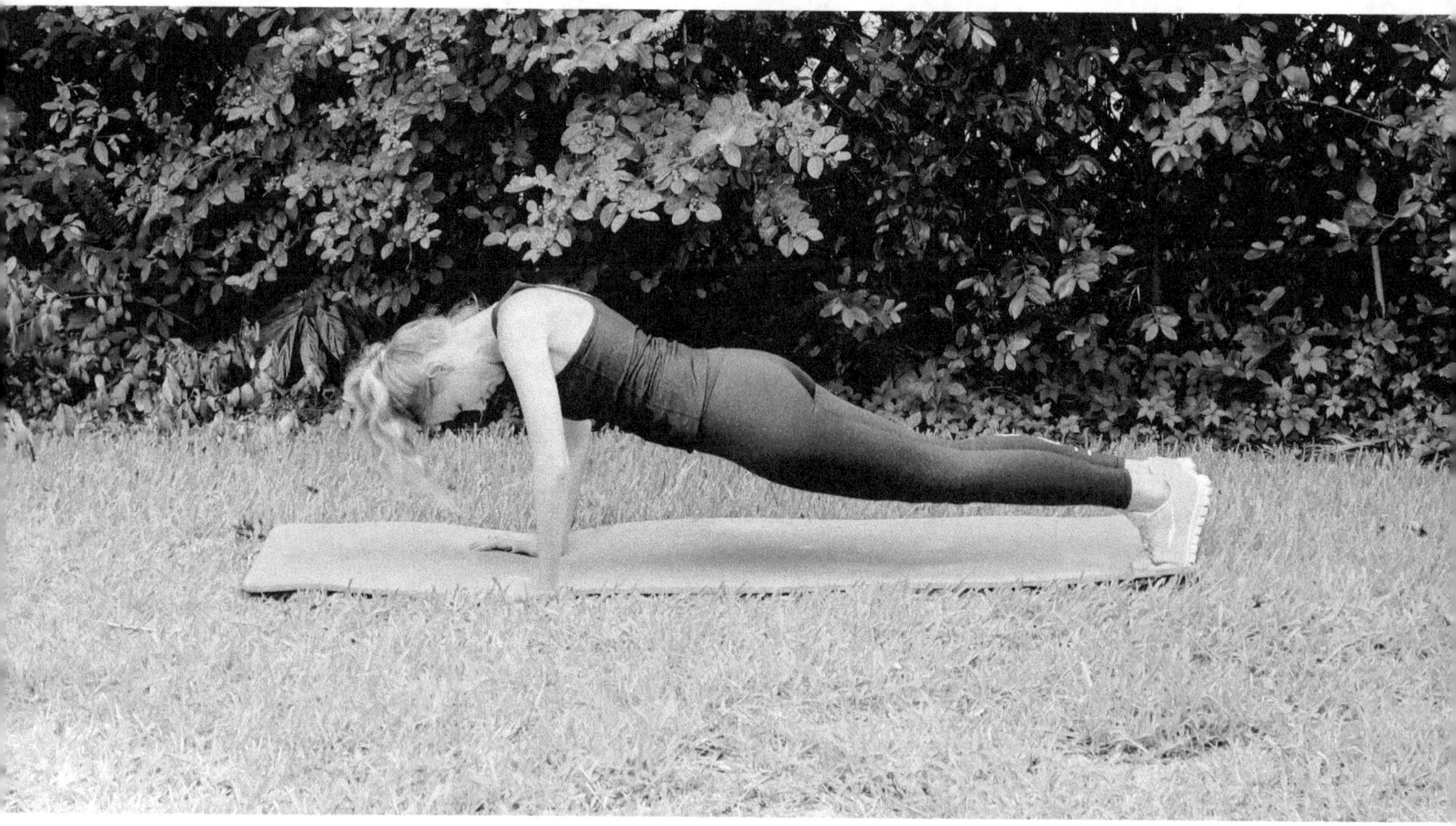

1. From a standing position, squat down and place your hands in front of you.

2. Kick back your feet into a push-up position, and then quickly bring them forward to land in a squat position.

3. Jump up so your feet leave the ground and repeat.

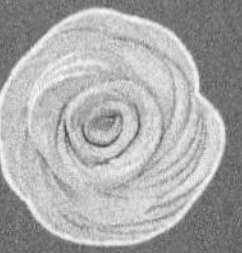

How to do Ice Skates

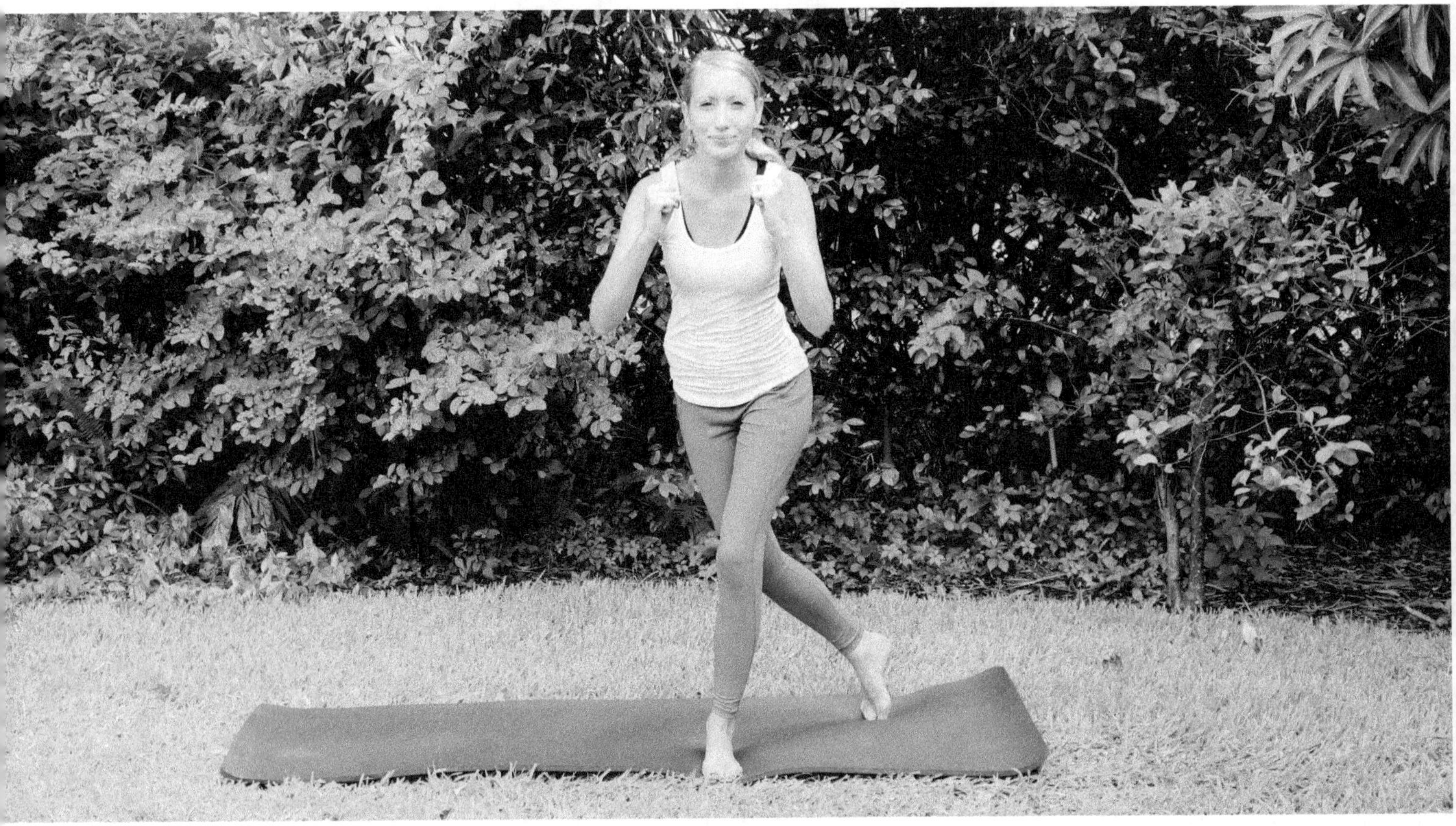

1. *Stand on left foot with right foot slightly lifted.*

2. *Jump as far as you can to the right, landing on your right foot, swinging your left foot behind your body.*

3. *Reverse the movement, jumping to the left, landing on your left foot, swinging your right foot behind your body.*

4. *Repeat.*

How to Jog In Place

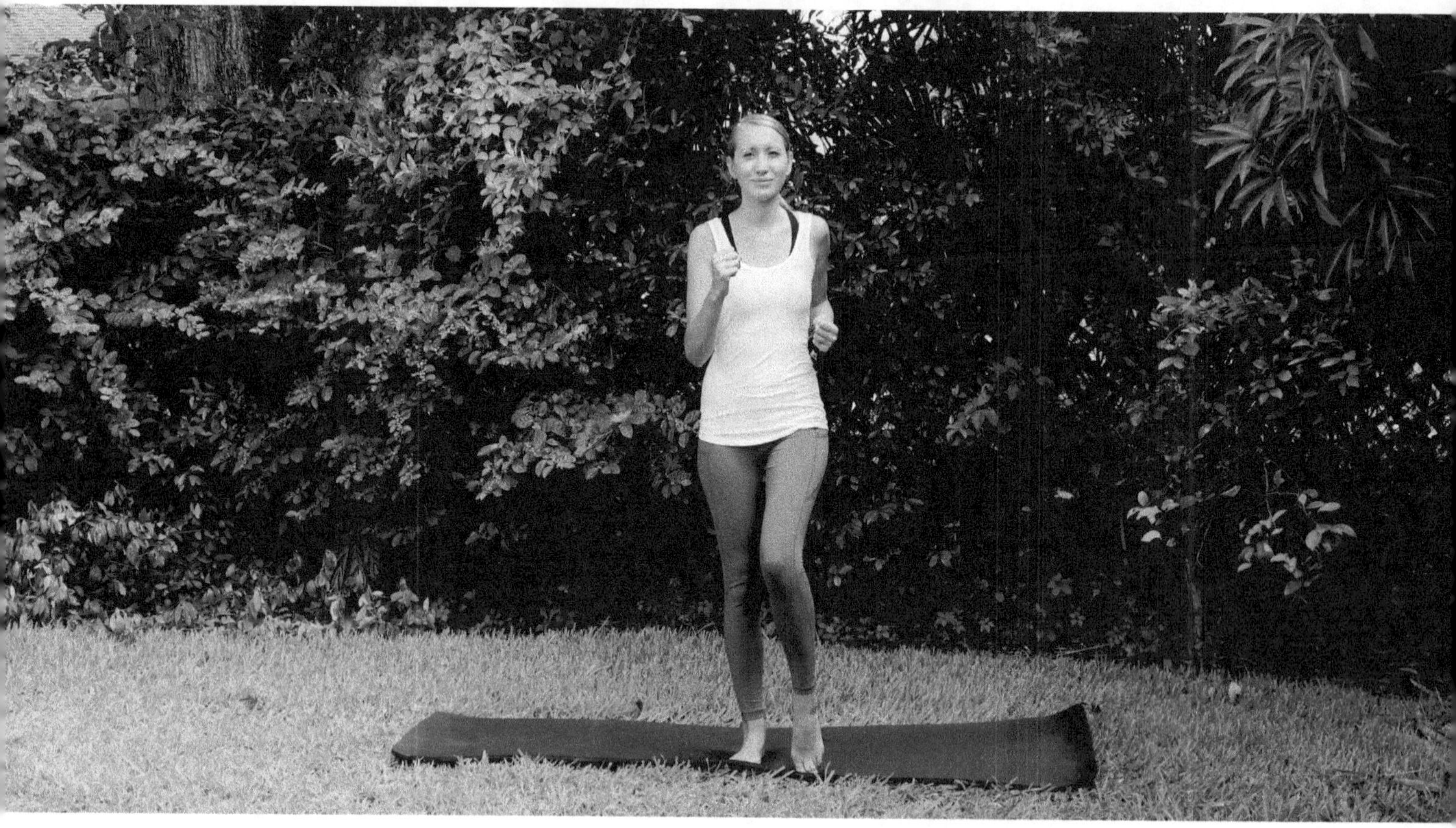

1. Start standing with your feet hip distance apart.

2. Lift one foot then the other to jog in place working your legs and increasing your heart rate.

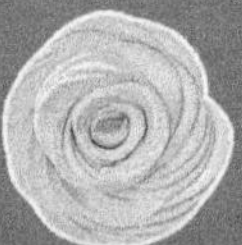

How to do Squats

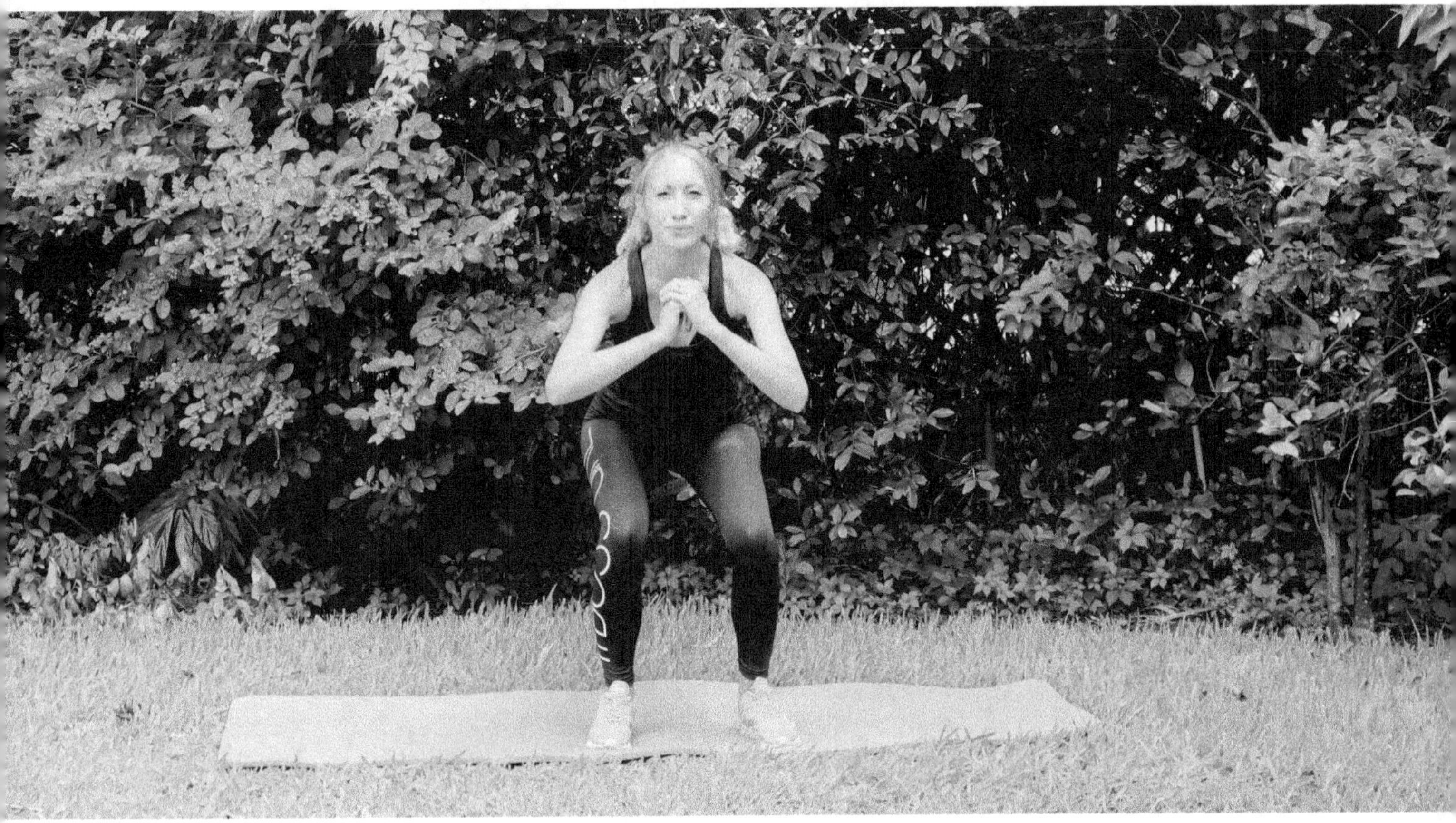

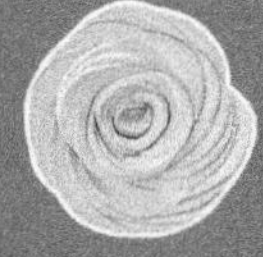

1. Stand with your head facing forward and your chest held up and out.Place your feet shoulder-width apart or slightly wider.

2. Bend your elbows and clasp your hands together.

3. Lower down so your thighs are as parallel to the floor as possible, with your knees over your ankles.

4. Press your weight back into your heels and keep your body tight.

5. Push through your heels to bring yourself back to the starting position and repeat.

How to do Boat Twists

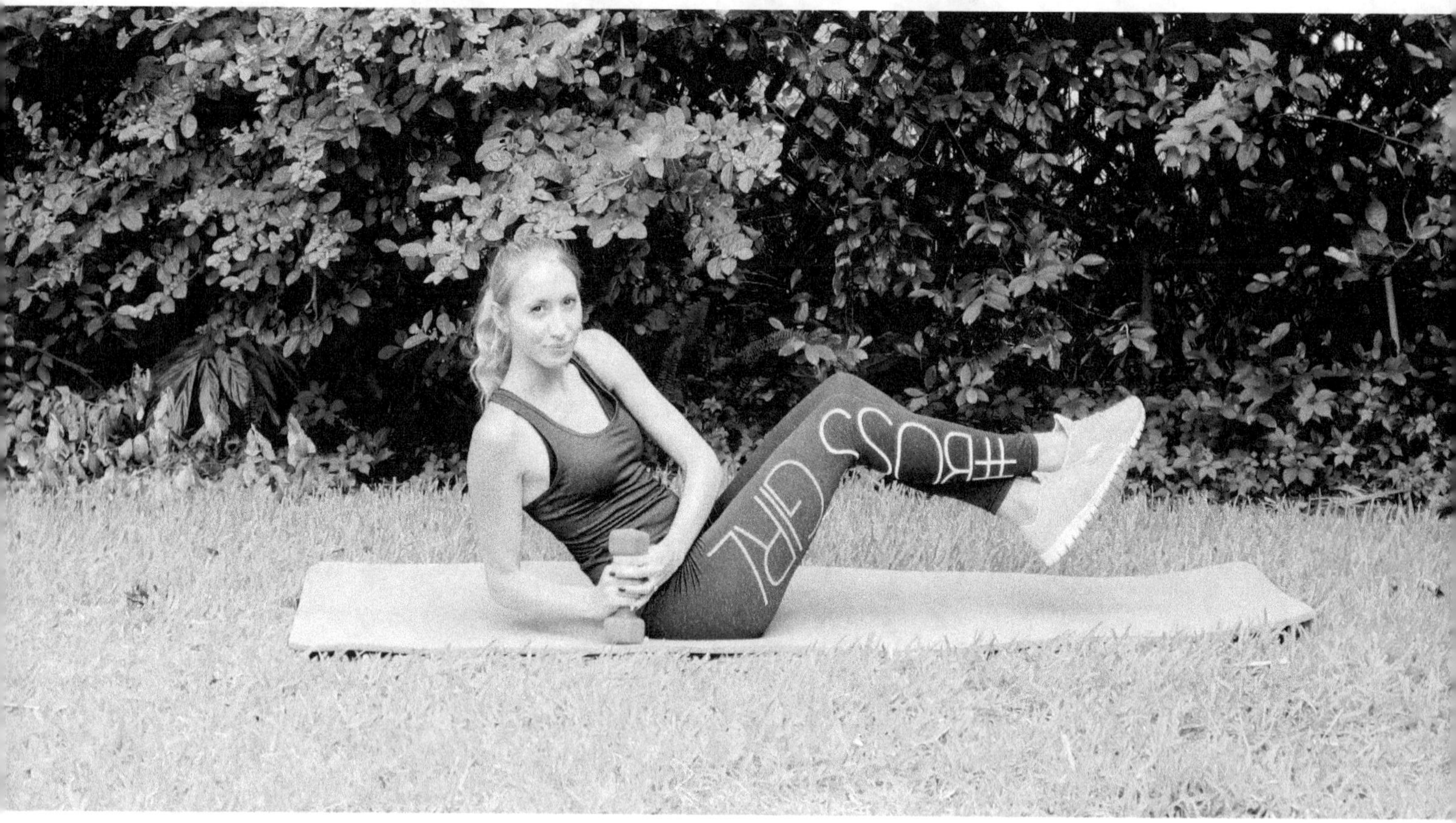

1. *Sit down on a mat with your knees bent while holding one dumbbell with both hands.*

2. *Extend your arms out to the sides and lift your feet off the floor.*

3. *Twist your torso and dumbbell to the right, and then reverse the motion, twisting it to the left.*

4. *Repeat.*

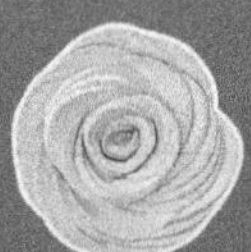

How to do Hollow Rocks

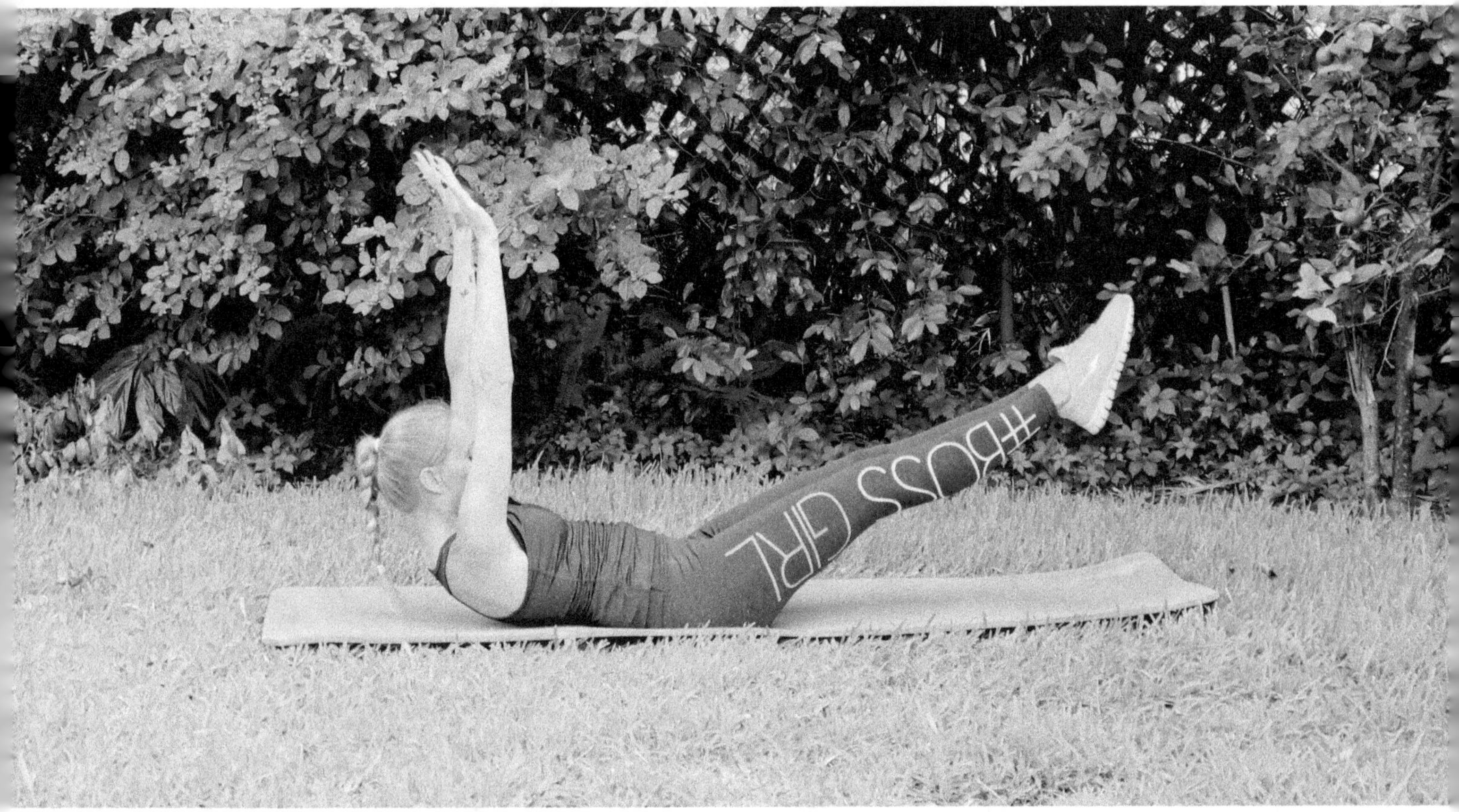

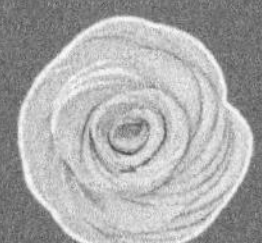

1. Lay down with your back on the ground and your arms straight back over your head.

2. Tighten up your core so that your lower back is flat against the mat.

3. Raise your feet and arms about 6 inches off of the ground.

4. While keeping your core tight begin to rock forward and backwards.

How to do Curtsy Lunges

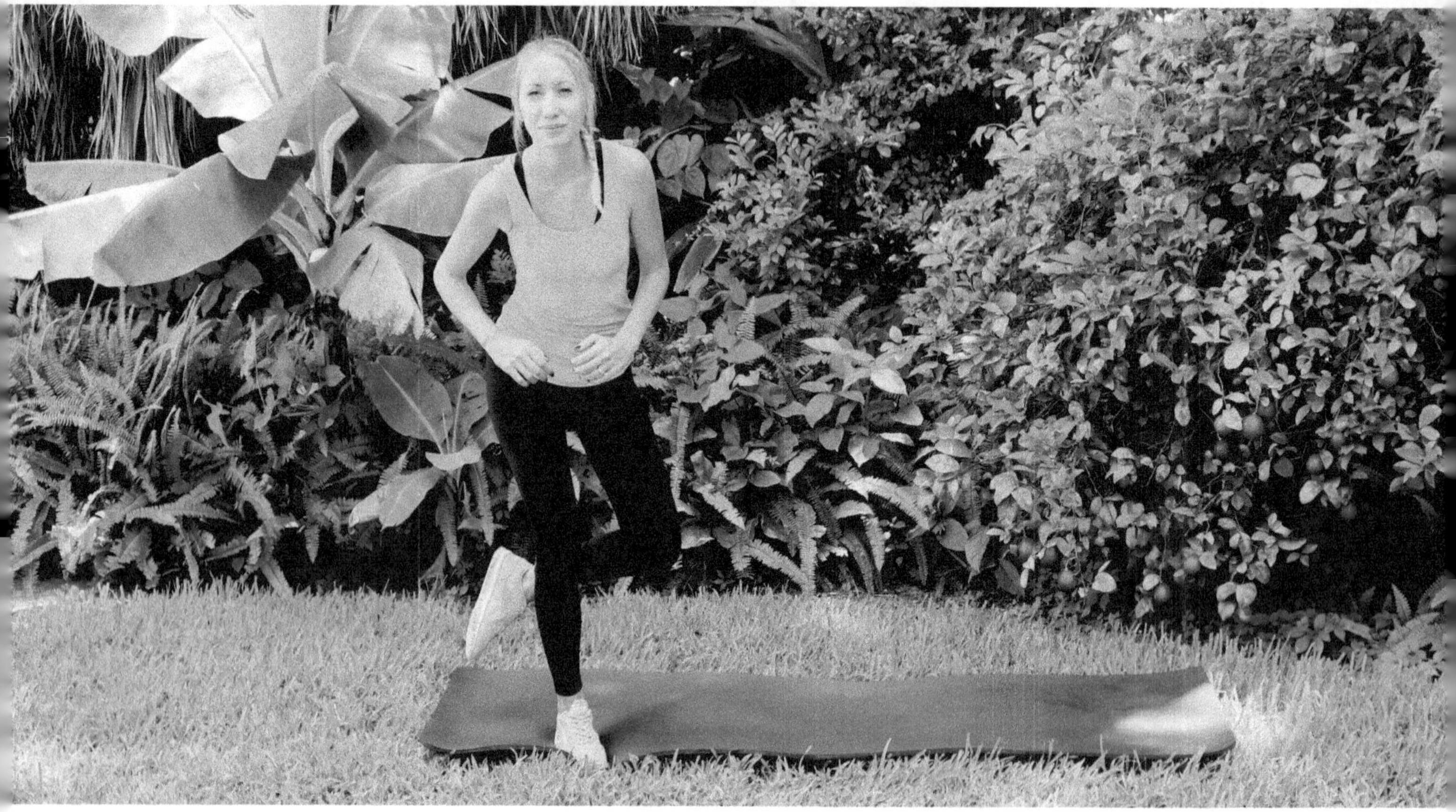

1. Stand with your feet hip-width apart.

2. Take a big step back with your left leg, crossing it behind your right.

3. Bend your knees and lower your hips until your right thigh is nearly parallel to the floor.

4. Keep your torso upright and your hips and shoulders as square as possible.

5. Return to start and repeat, stepping back with your right leg.

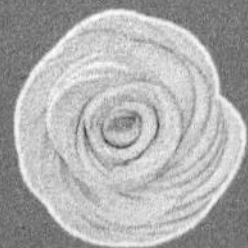

How to do Step-Ups

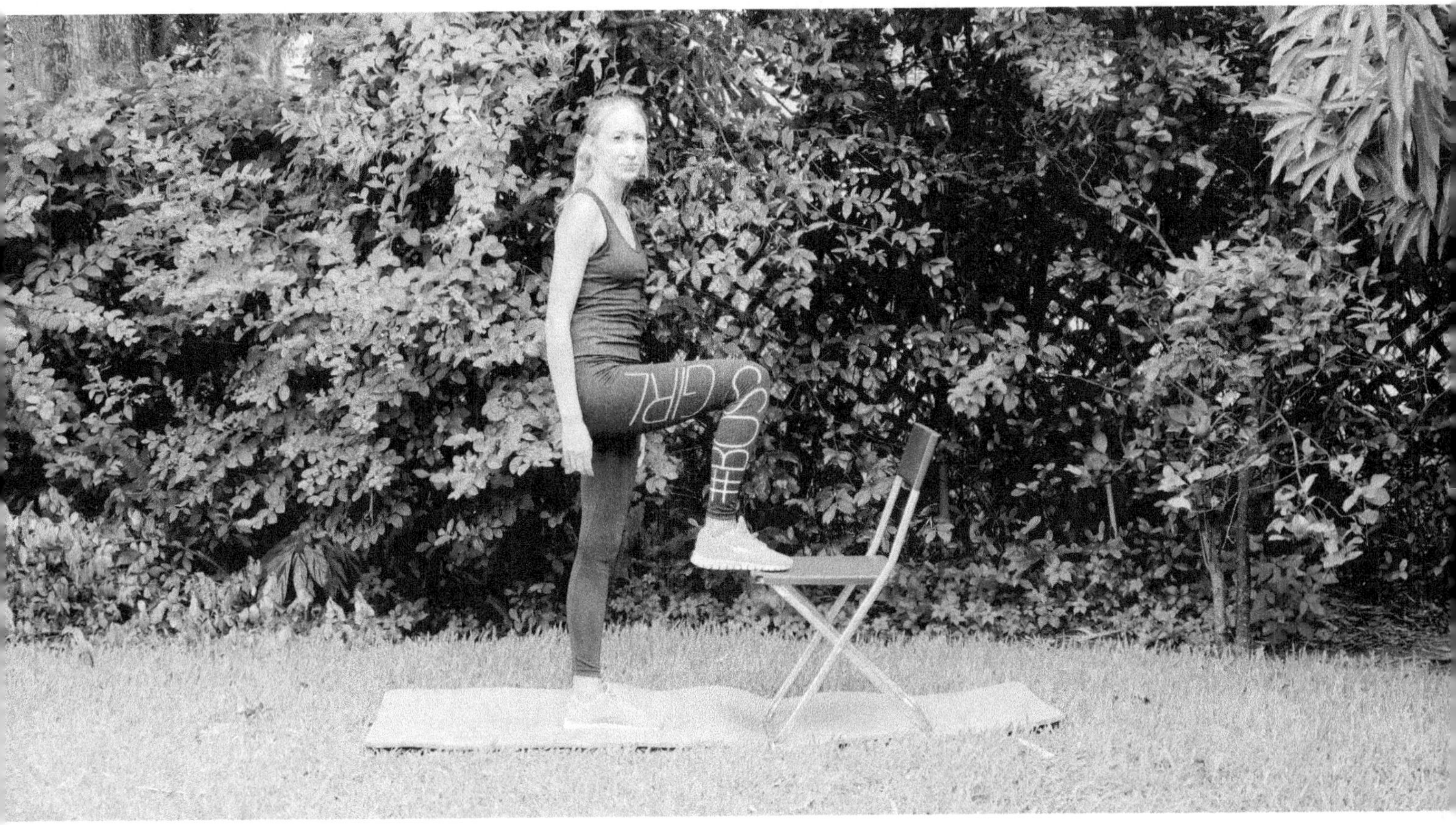

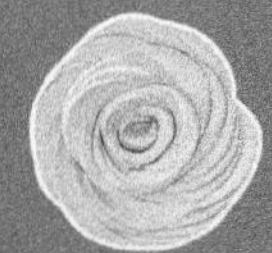

1. *Place your entire right foot onto the bench or chair.*

2. *Press through your right heel as you step onto the bench, bringing your left foot to meet your right foot so you are standing on the bench.*

3. *Return to the starting position by stepping down with the right foot, then the left so both feet are on the floor.*

4. *Repeat with alternating each leg.*

How to do Dumbbell Thrusters

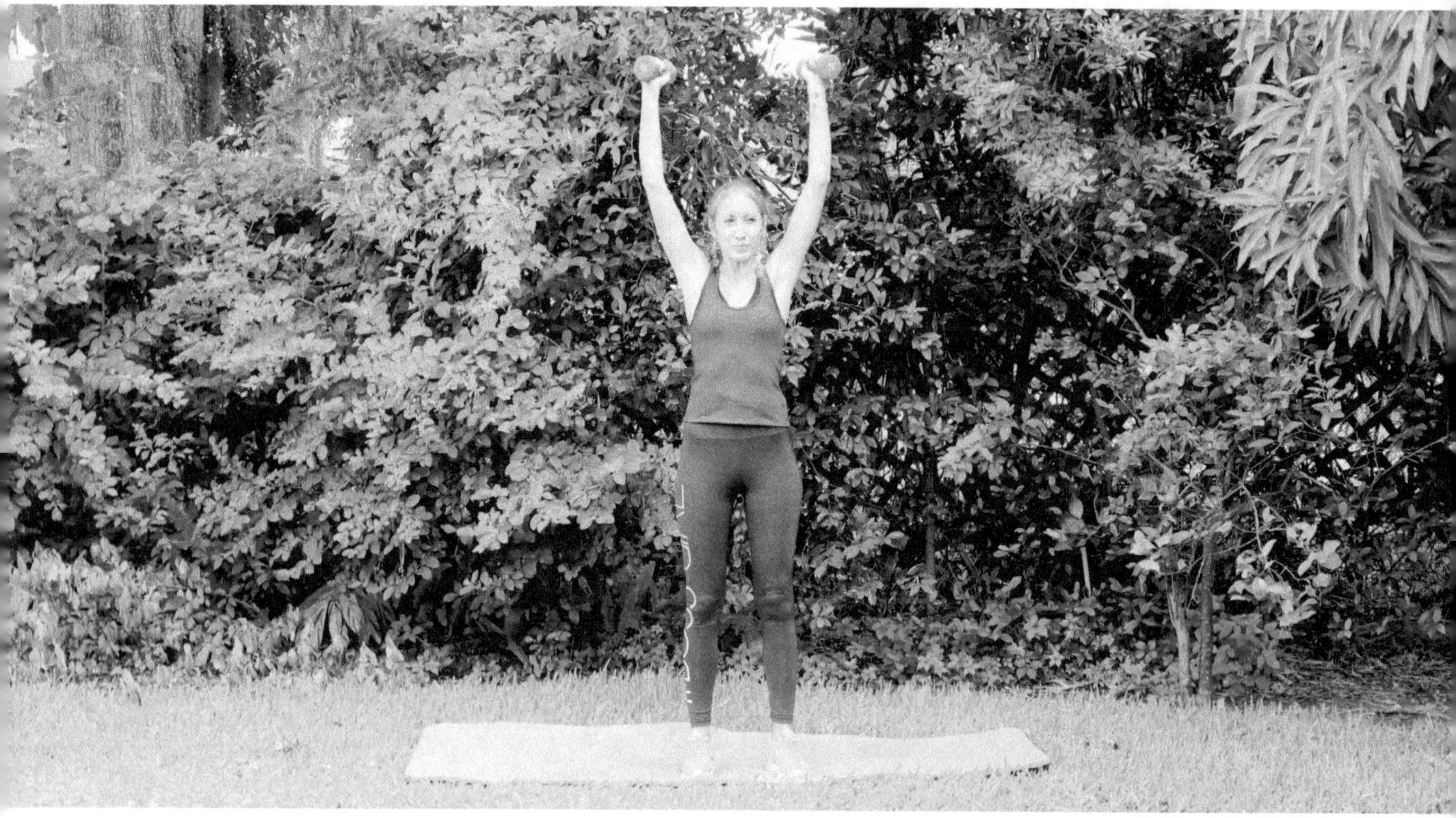

1. *Assume a slightly wider than shoulder width stance and hold two dumbbells to your shoulders with a neutral grip.*

2. *Inhale and complete a normal front squat with dumbbells in place by simultaneously flexing the knees and hips together.*

3. *Press your whole foot into the floor and extend the legs.*

4. *As you return to the starting position, utilize your momentum from the front squat to propel the dumbbells upward into a push press.*

5. *Exhale once the dumbbells get to lockout and reverse the movement slowly while controlling them back to your shoulders.*

6. *Repeat.*

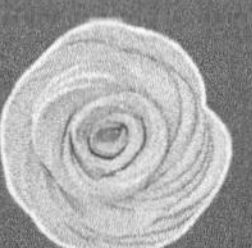

How to do Dumbbell Rows

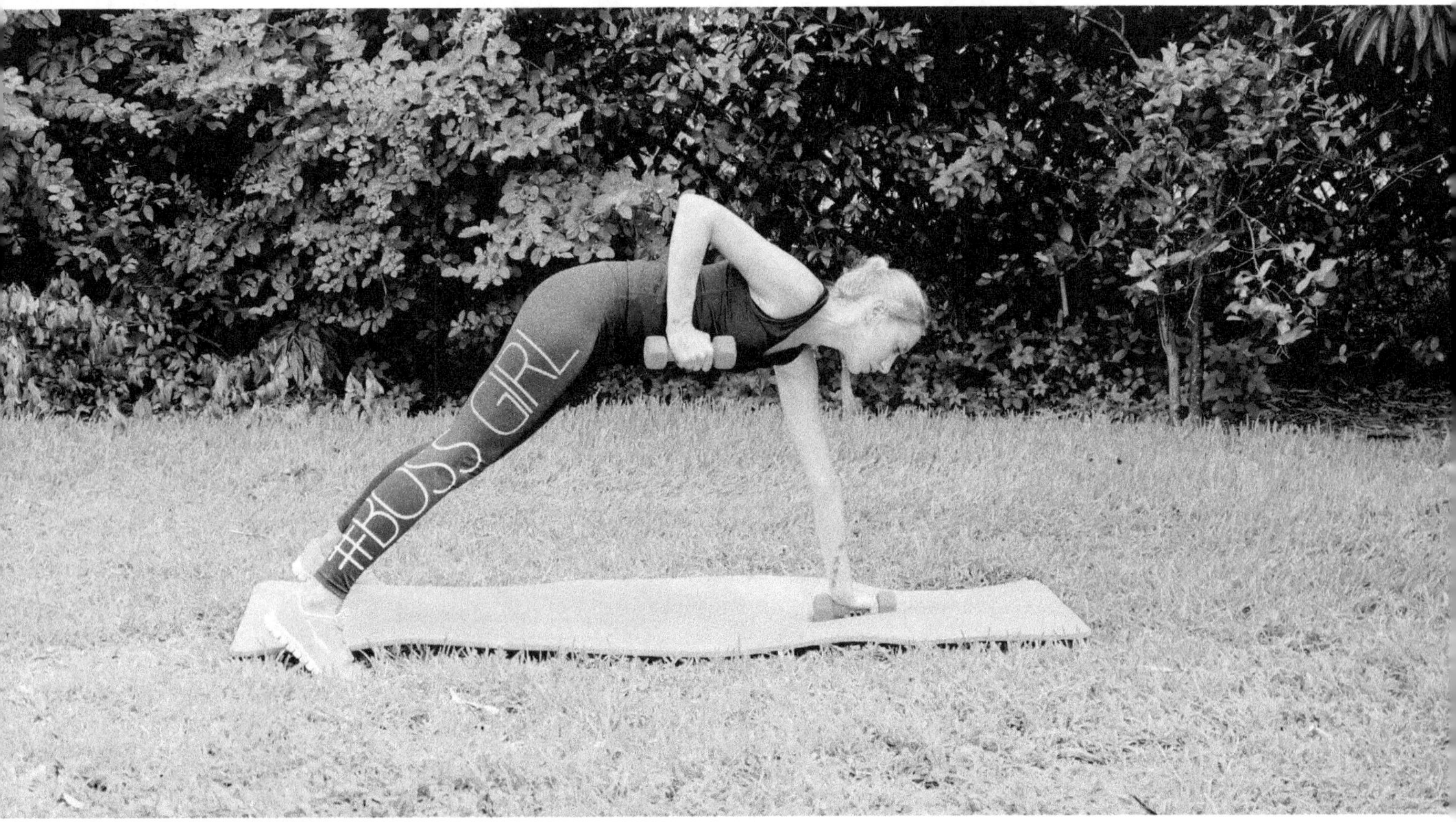

1. Grab a pair of dumbbells, bend at your hips and knees, and lower your torso until it's almost parallel to the floor.

2. Let the weights hang at arm's length from your shoulders.

3. Pull your shoulders down and back and hold that position.

4. Then pull the weight to the side of your ribs by squeezing your shoulder blades toward your spine. Hold it for a bit.

5. Lower the weight to the starting position and repeat.

6. Then repeat on opposite side.

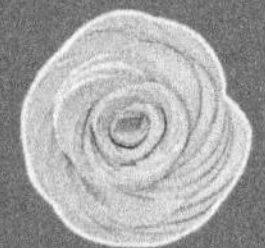

How to do Downward-Facing Dog

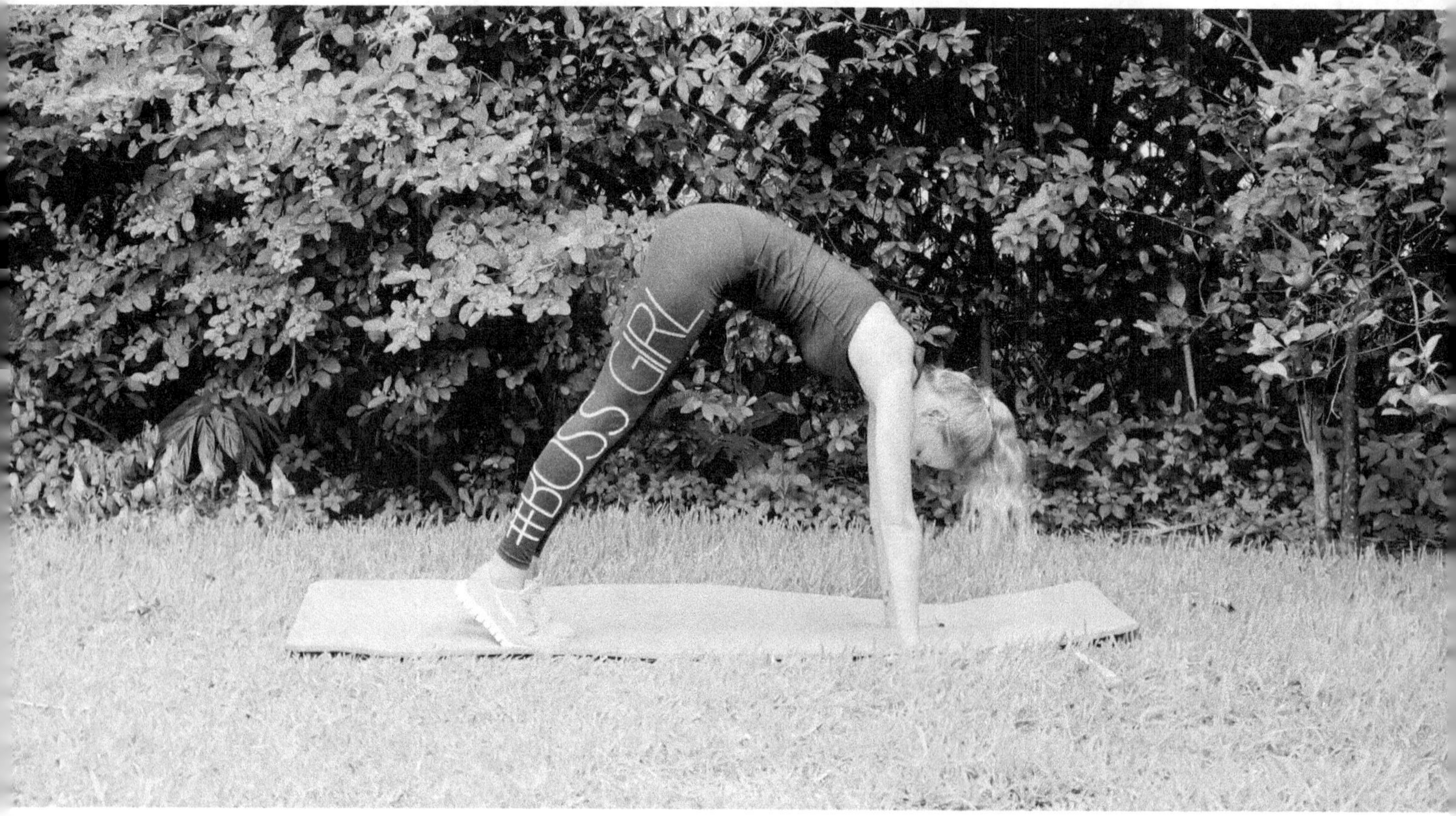

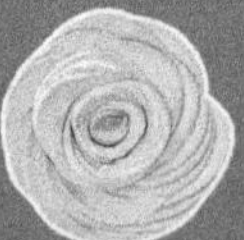

1. *Begin in a kneeling position on your mat with hands directly under shoulders, fingers spread wide.*

2. *Tuck your toes under and engage your abdominals as you push your body up off the mat so only your hands and feet are on the mat.*

3. *Press through your hands moving your chest gently toward your thighs and each heel alternating gently toward the floor.*

4. *Relax your head and neck and breathe fully.*

How to Run On The Spot With High Knees

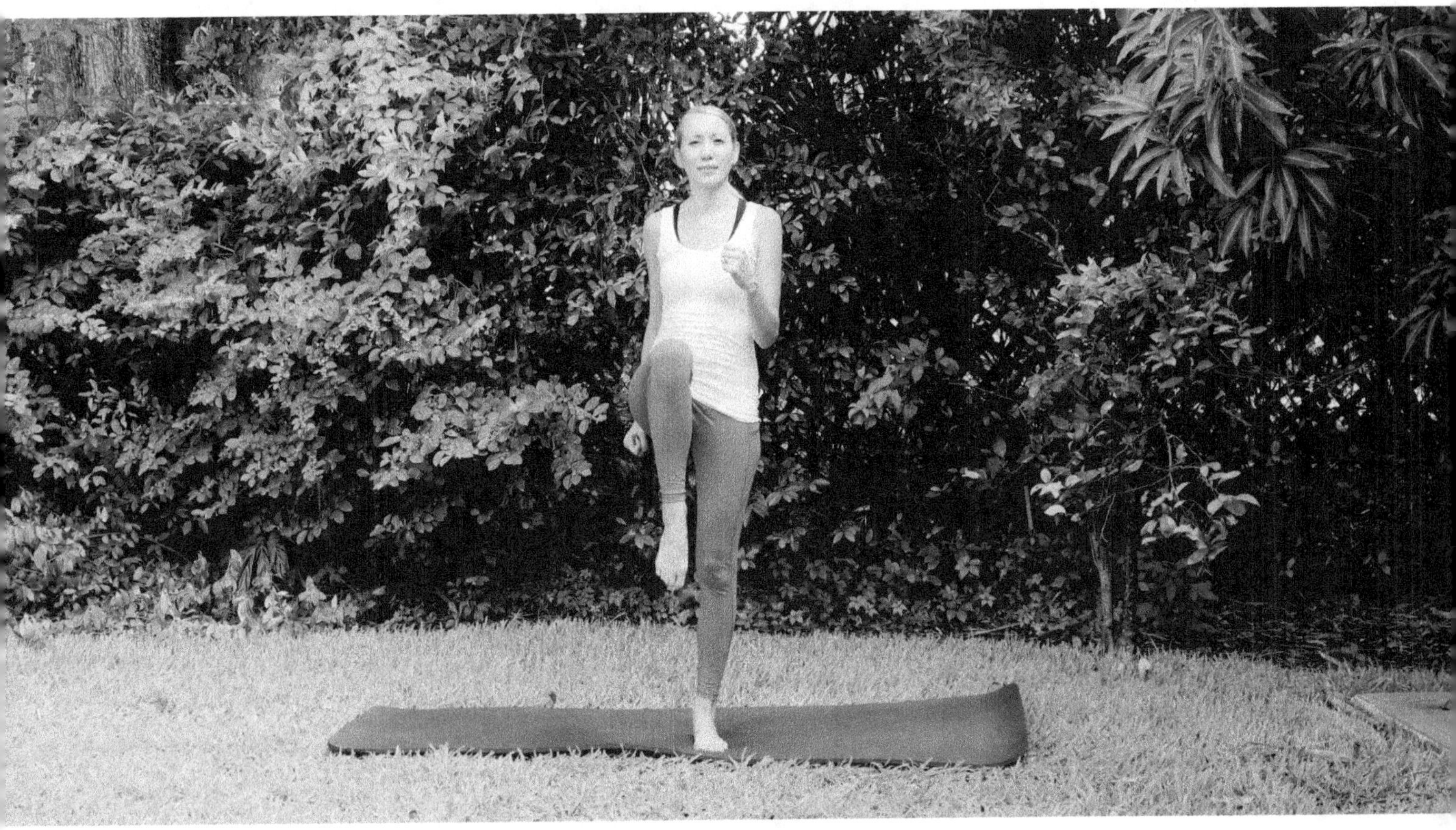

1. *Start by running in place, raising your knees up high.*

2. *Arms pumping back and forth.*

3. *Continue for the desired time.*

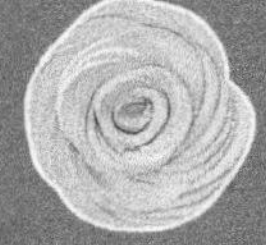

How to do Resistance Band Donkey Kicks

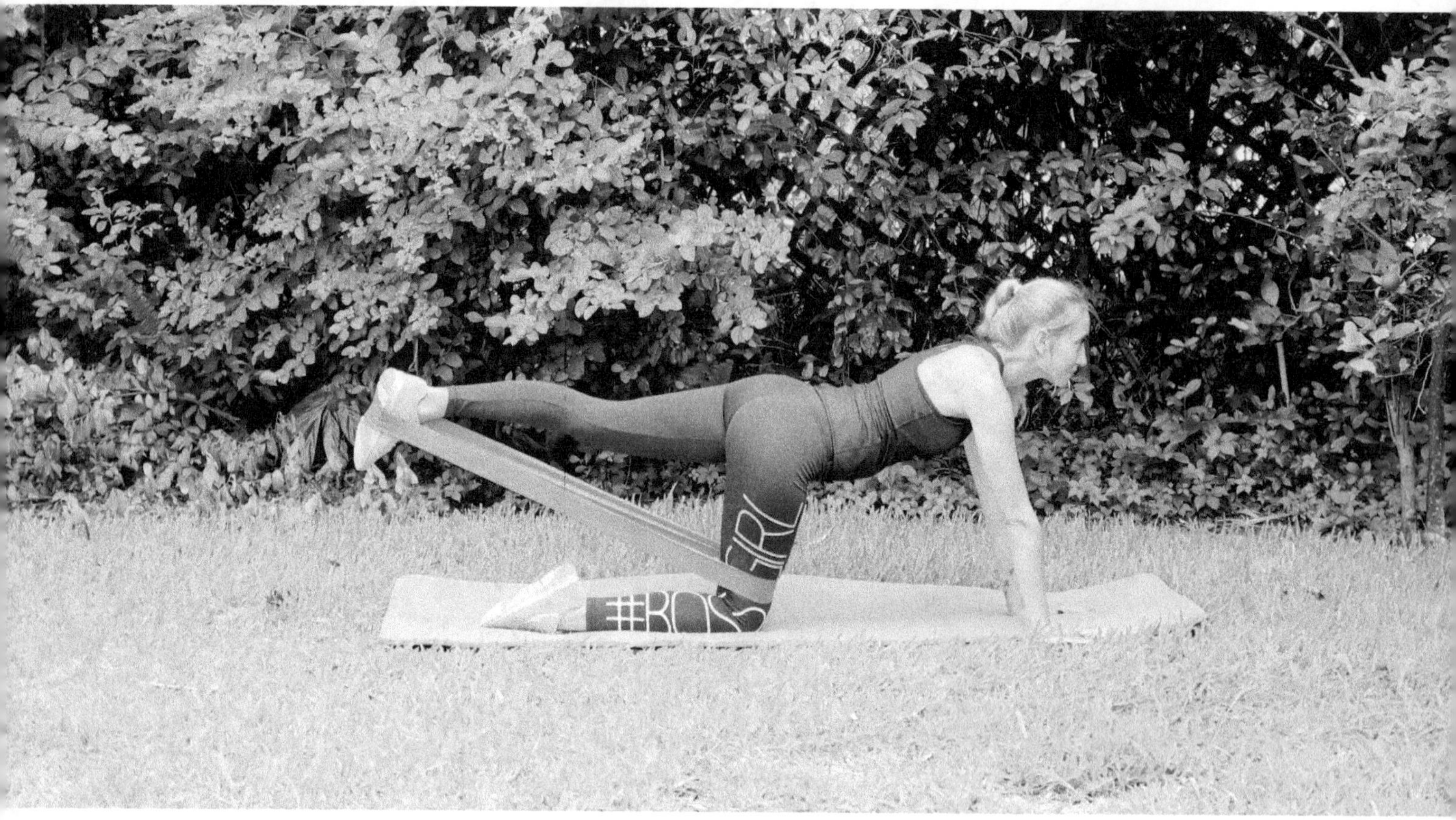

1. Put the one end of the resistance band around your thigh.

2. Position your hands so they are directly under your face, elbows straight.

3. Hook your right foot into the band on the other end.

4. Keeping your back straight, push your right leg out and up.

5. Draw it back and repeat.

6. Alternate sides.

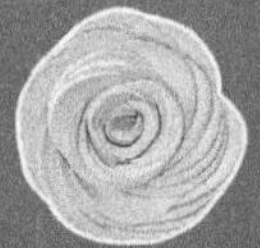

How to do Fire Hydrant

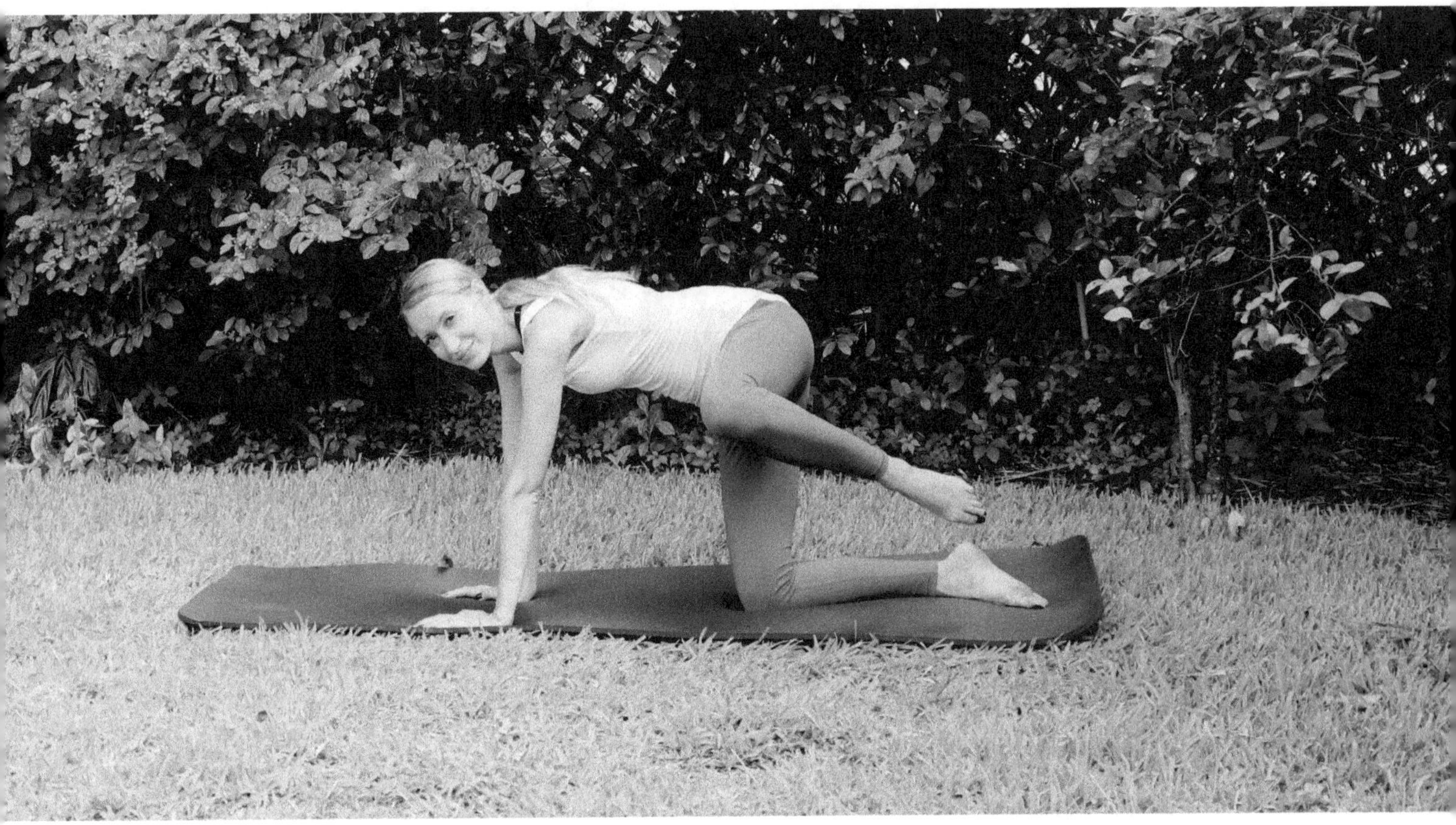

1. *Start on all-fours, aligning your shoulders over your wrists and your knees directly underneath your hips while keeping your spine long and neutral.*

2. *Lift your right knee to the right while keeping the rest of your body still, then lower it back to the ground with control.*

3. *Repeat.*

4. *Alternate to other side.*

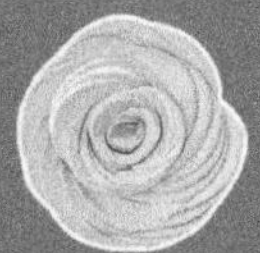

How to do Fire Hydrant With a Circle

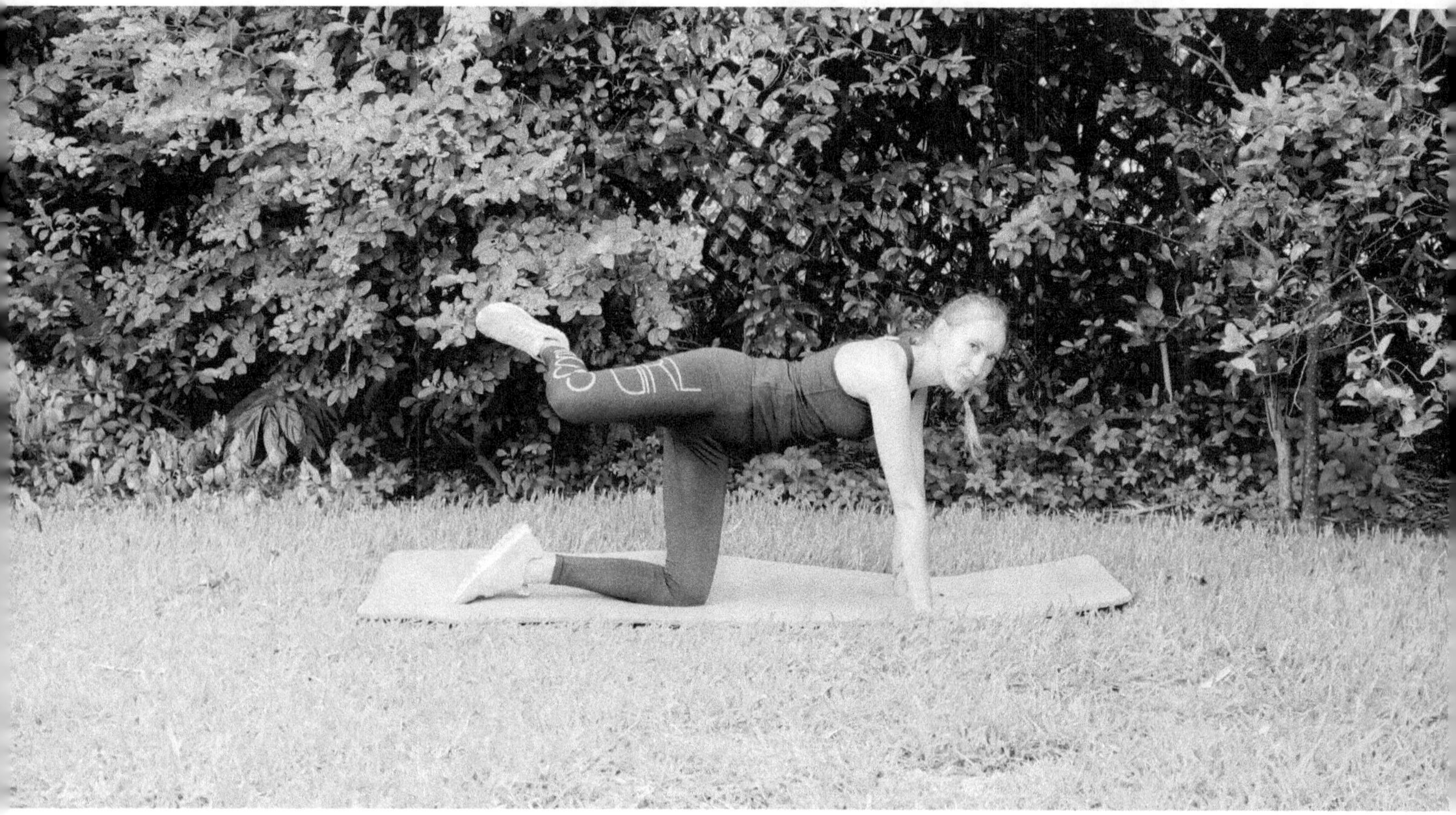

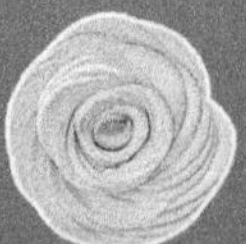

1. Start on all fours with your hands directly under your shoulders and your knees directly under your hips.

2. Moving from your hip, lift your left knee up off of the ground. From here draw and imaginary semicircle with your left knee, slightly opening your hip, moving your knee forward.

3. Complete the motion by bringing your left knee back underneath your left hip.

4. Repeat and then alternate sides.

How to do V Sit-Ups

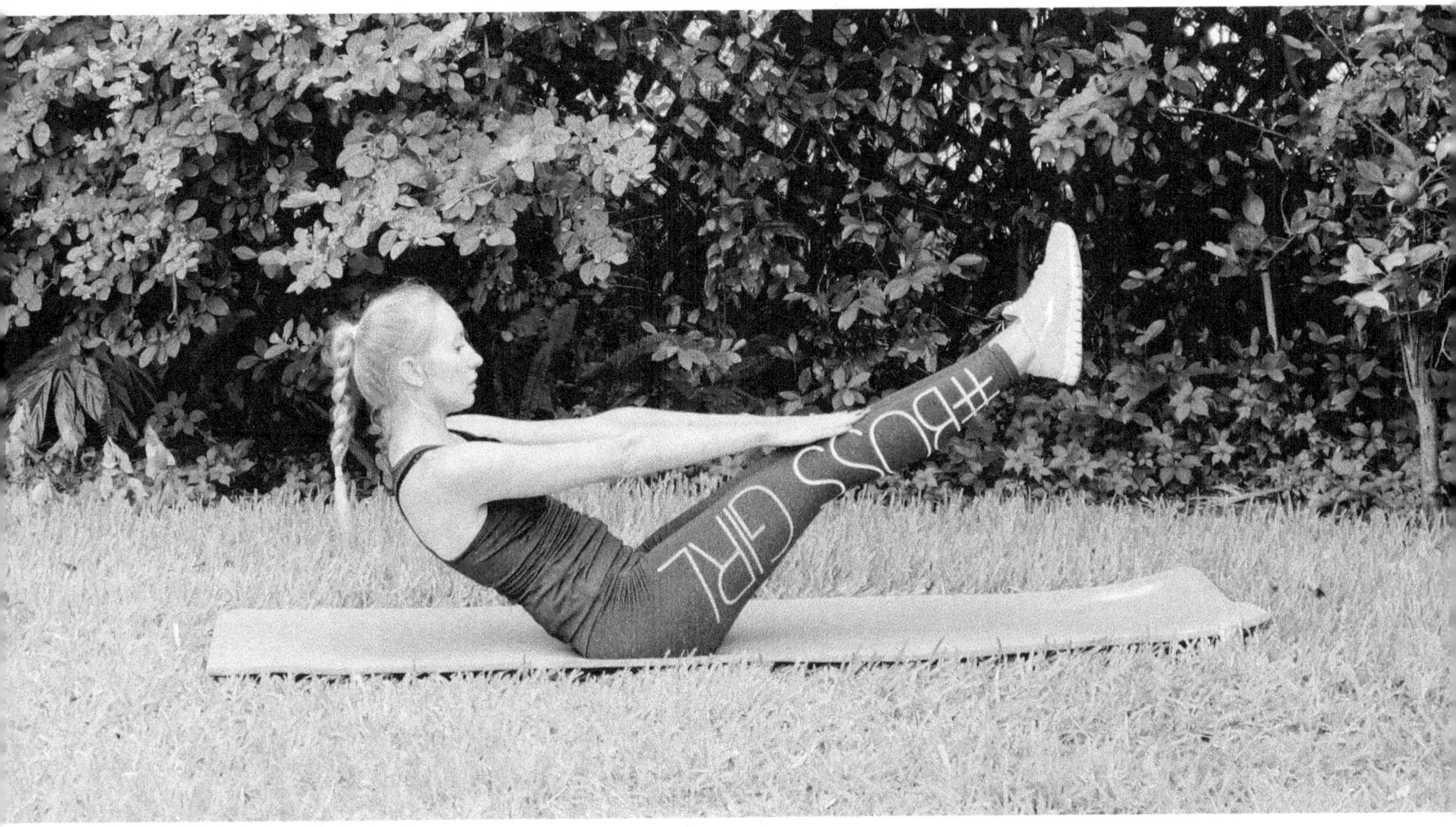

1. *Begin on your back with your arms extended over your head and your legs straight out on the ground.*

2. *Pull your arms forward while you lift your shoulders off of the ground.*

3. *At the same time, keep your lower back on the ground and pull your legs upwards to meet your arms. Pause and gently lower back to the ground.*

4. *Repeat.*

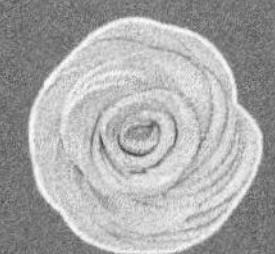

Simple Lightweight Dumbbell Workouts

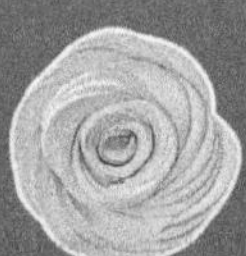

How to do Goblet Squats

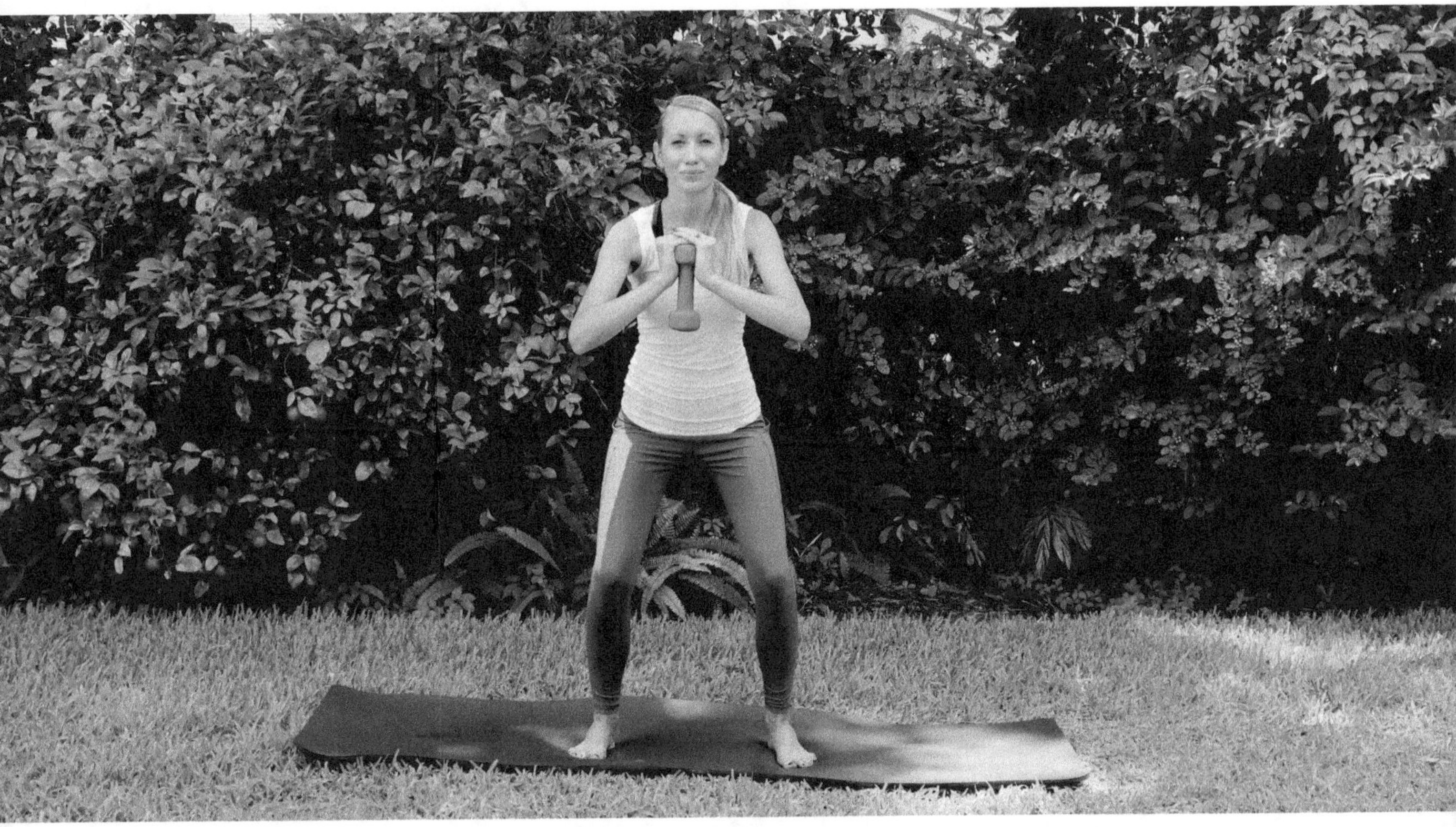

1. Hold a weight at your chest in both hands, elbows close to your body, and stand with your feet slightly wider than hip-width apart.

2. Bend your knees and drop your butt back and down to lower into a squat. Keep your chest high and core tight.

3. Push your knees out and make sure to keep the weight in your heels.

4. Push through your heels to stand back up, and squeeze your glutes at the top and repeat.

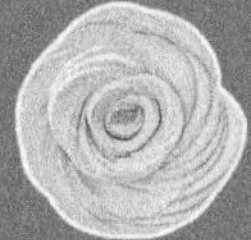

How to do Shoulder Presses

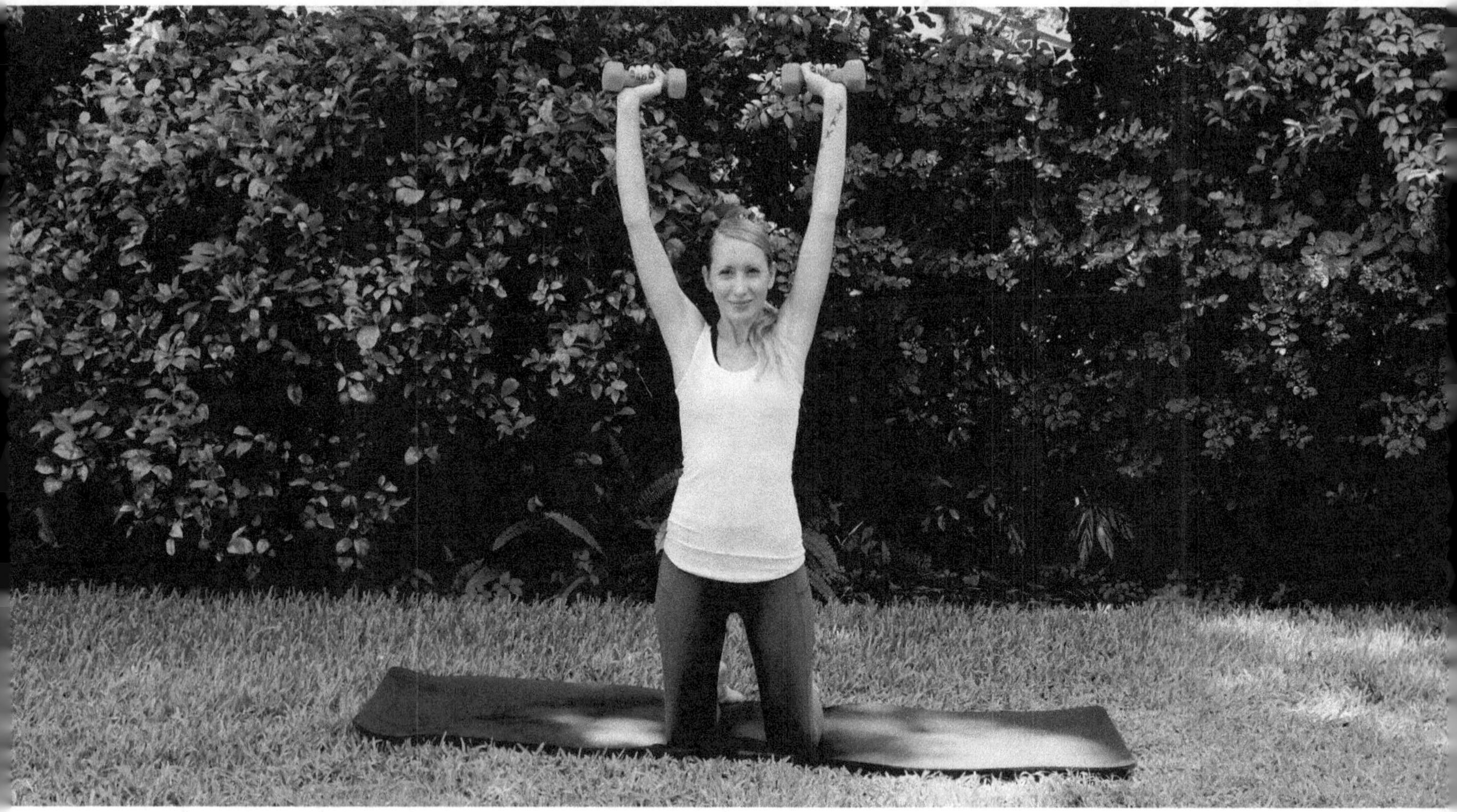

1. Stand with your feet slightly wider than hip-width apart, or kneel with your back straight and core tight.

2. Hold a pair of dumbbells and start with you arms raised to shoulder-height, elbows bent so the weights are in the air. Rotate your wrists so your palms are facing forward.

3. Press the dumbbells overhead. Keep your elbows facing forward during the press.

4. Pause at the top once your arms are fully extended. Then, slowly return the weights to starting position and repeat.

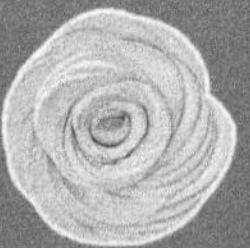

How to do Basic Stiff-Leg Deadlifts

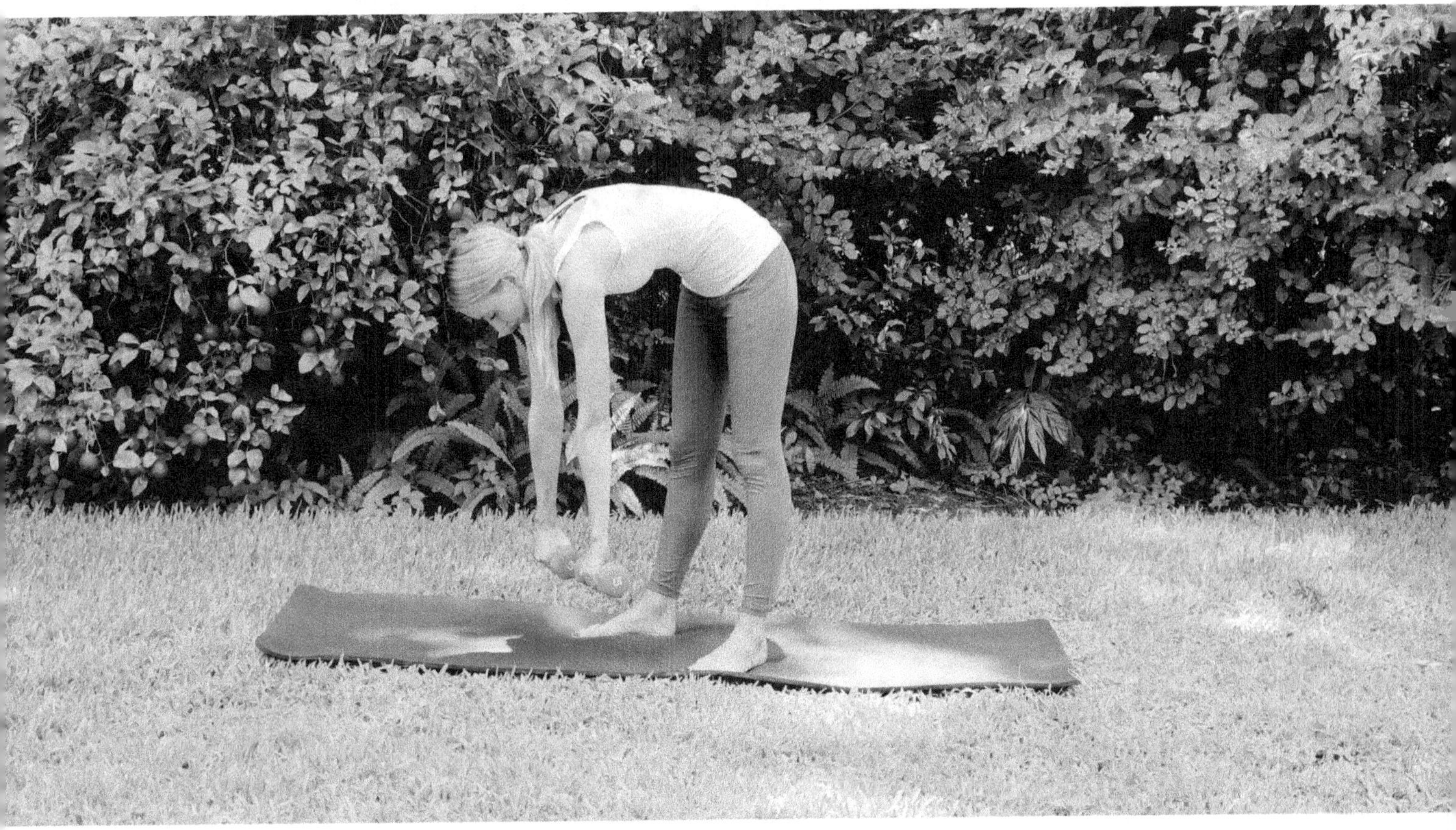

1. *Stand with feet hip-width apart, knees slightly bent, holding a dumbbell in each hand.*

2. *Hinge at your hips and bend your knees slightly as you lower your body. Think about pushing your butt back.*

3. *Hold the dumbbells close to your legs as you descend. Pull back on your shoulder blades and do not let your back arch.*

4. *Keeping your core tight, push through your heels to stand up straight. Keep the weights close to your shins as you pull.*

5. *Pause at the top and squeeze your butt to complete and repeat.*

How to do Bent-Over Rows

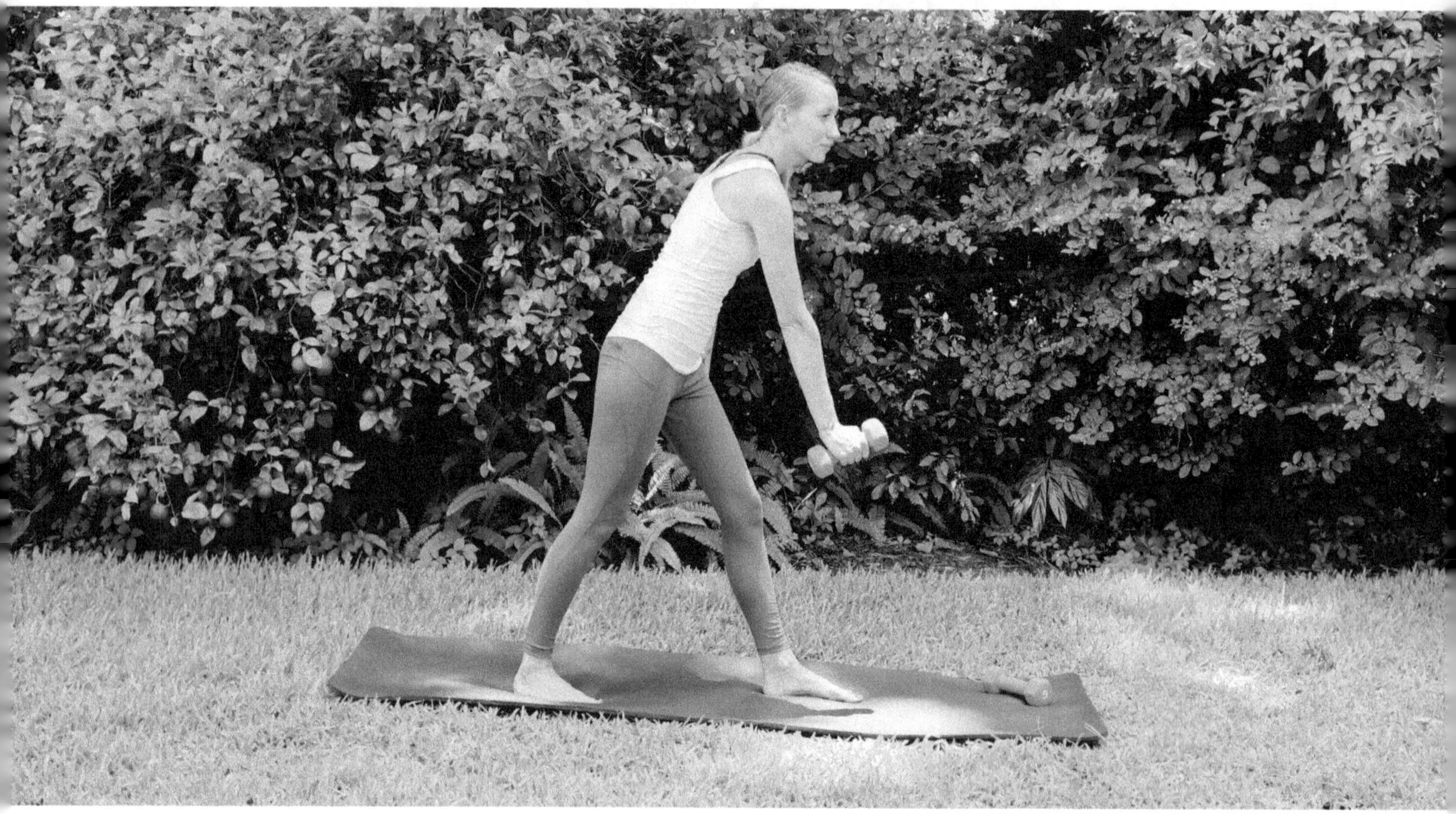

1. *Hold a dumbbell in one hand. Step the opposite leg forward so that you're standing in a staggered stance. Hinge forward at the hips so your torso is angled toward the floor and your back is flat.*

2. *Keeping your body in this position, lift the dumbbell up to chest level, keeping your elbow close to your side.*

3. *In a controlled motion, lower the dumbbell back down to the starting position and repeat.*

4. *Then repeat on opposite side.*

www.ketoveo.com

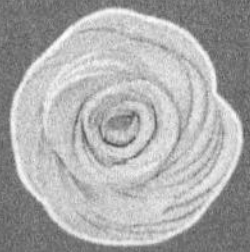

How to do Chest Presses

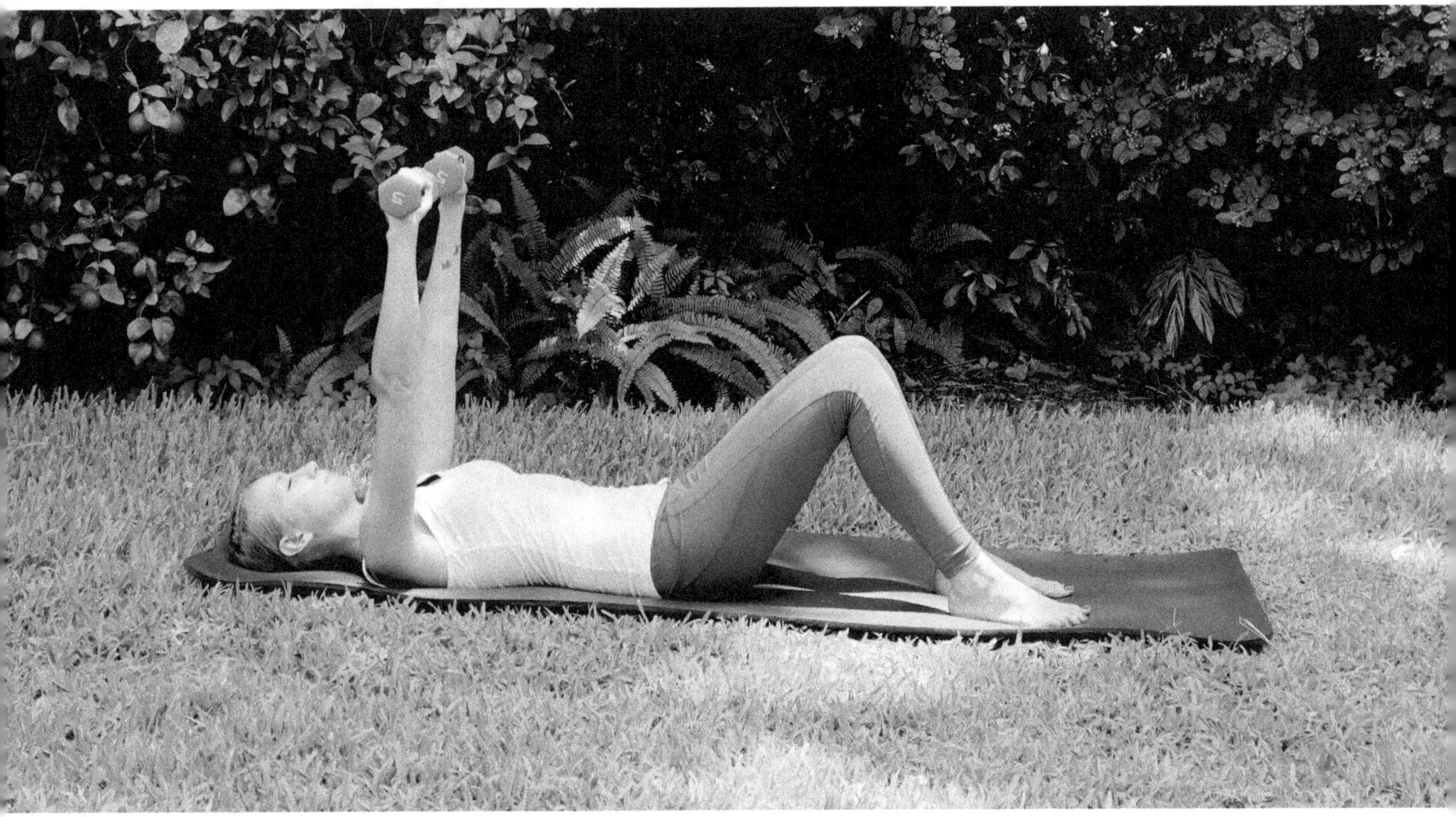

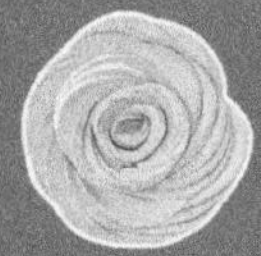

1. *Lie on your back on the floor or on a flat bench, holding a dumbbell in each hand.*

2. *Rotate your wrists forward so that the palms of your hands are facing away from you.*

3. *Hold the dumbbells at the sides of your chest, elbows bent at a 90-degree angle.*

4. *Press the dumbbells up and together. Think about using your chest muscles to initiate the movement.*

5. *Bring your arms back down to starting position and repeat.*

How to do Glute Bridges

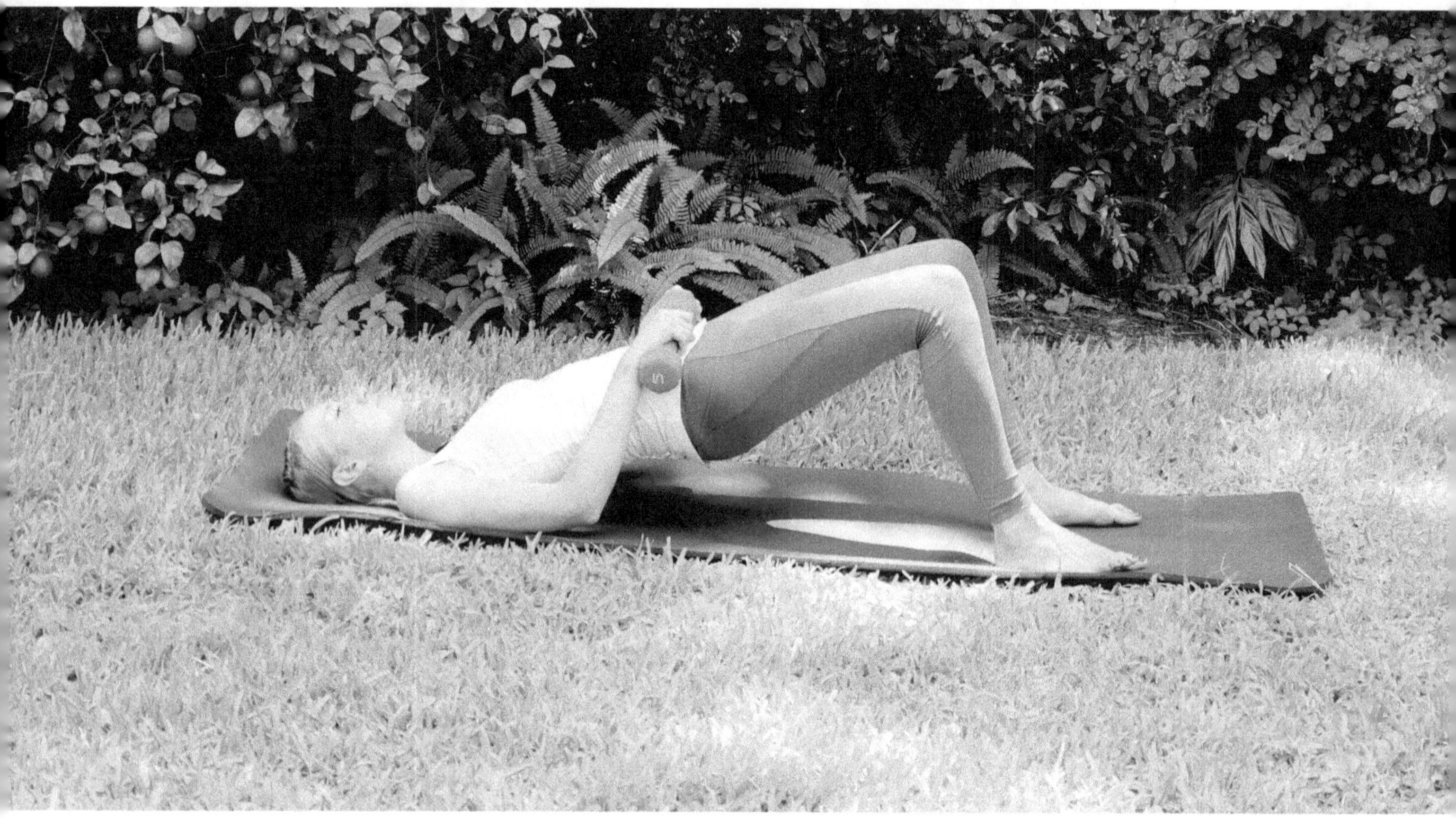

1. Lie on your back with your knees bent, feet flat on the floor, and dumbbells resting on your hips. Your feet should be about hip-distance apart with your heels a few inches away from your butt.

1. Push through your heels to lift your hips up while squeezing your glutes. Try to create one diagonal line from your shoulders to your knees.

1. Pause for 1 to 2 seconds, then slowly lower back down to the ground and repeat.

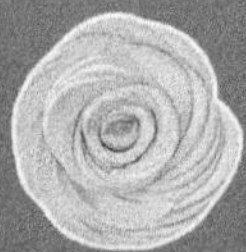

Resistance Band With Handle Workouts

How to do Lunges

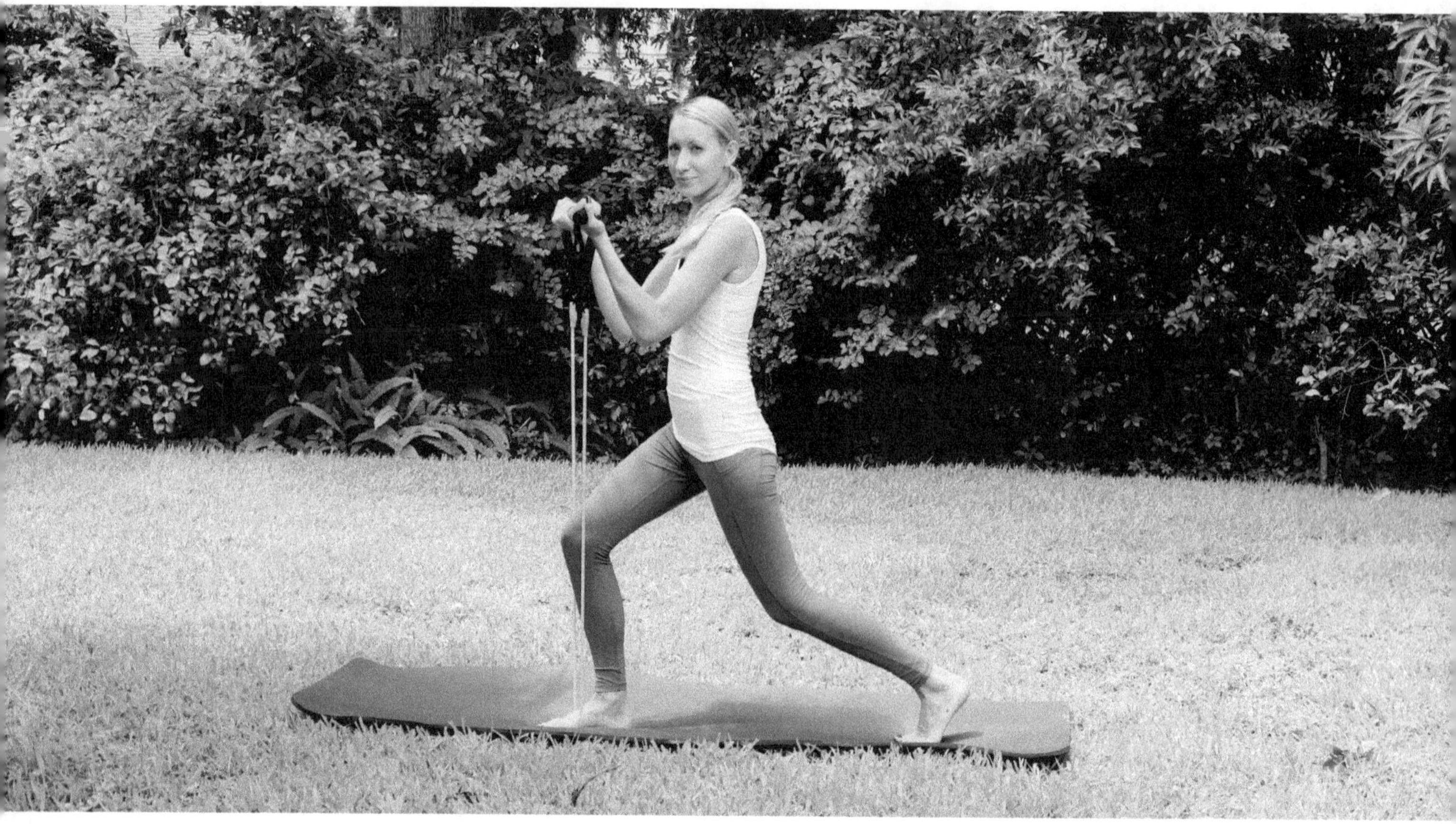

1. *Stand in a staggered stance and position your front foot on top of the cable with your back foot slightly behind your body and knees slightly bent.*

2. *Grasp the handles and position them at shoulder height in front of you.*

3. *Bend your legs, keeping your back knee above the floor and your front knee over your toes.*

4. *Keep your shoulder blades squeezed together, and your head and chest forward.*

5. *Push back up to start and repeat.*

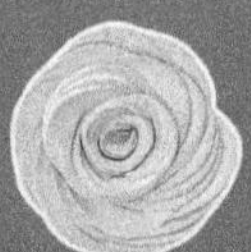

How to do Front Raises

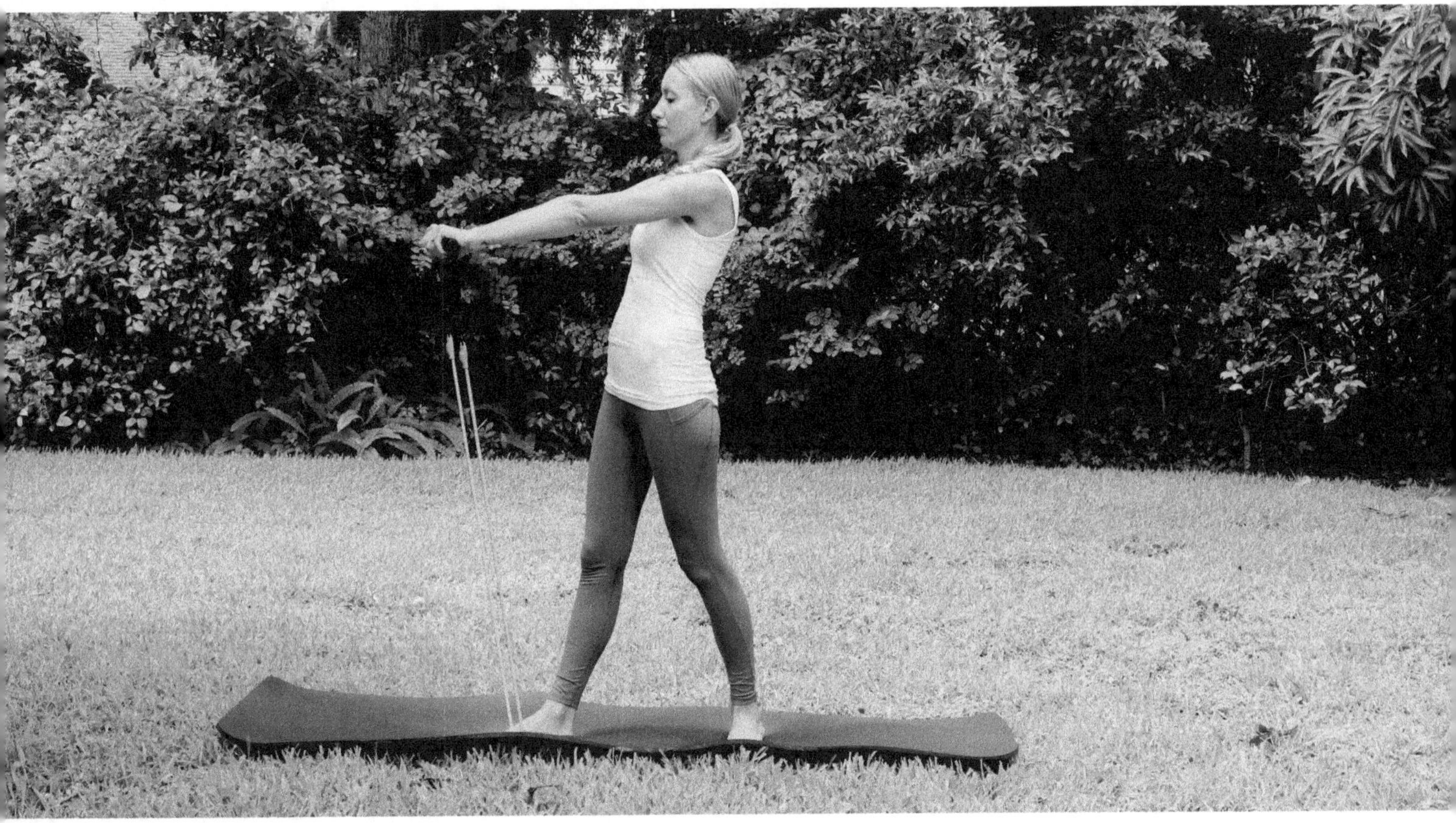

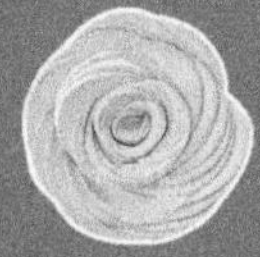

1. *Stand in a staggered stance. Place cable under your front foot with your knees slightly bent.*

2. *Grasp the handles with your palms facing your thighs and position your arms on the sides of your body directly under your shoulders.*

3. *Lift your arms up and forward in front of your shoulders.*

4. *Keep wrists firm and elbows soft.*

5. *Return to start and repeat.*

How to do Chest Flyes

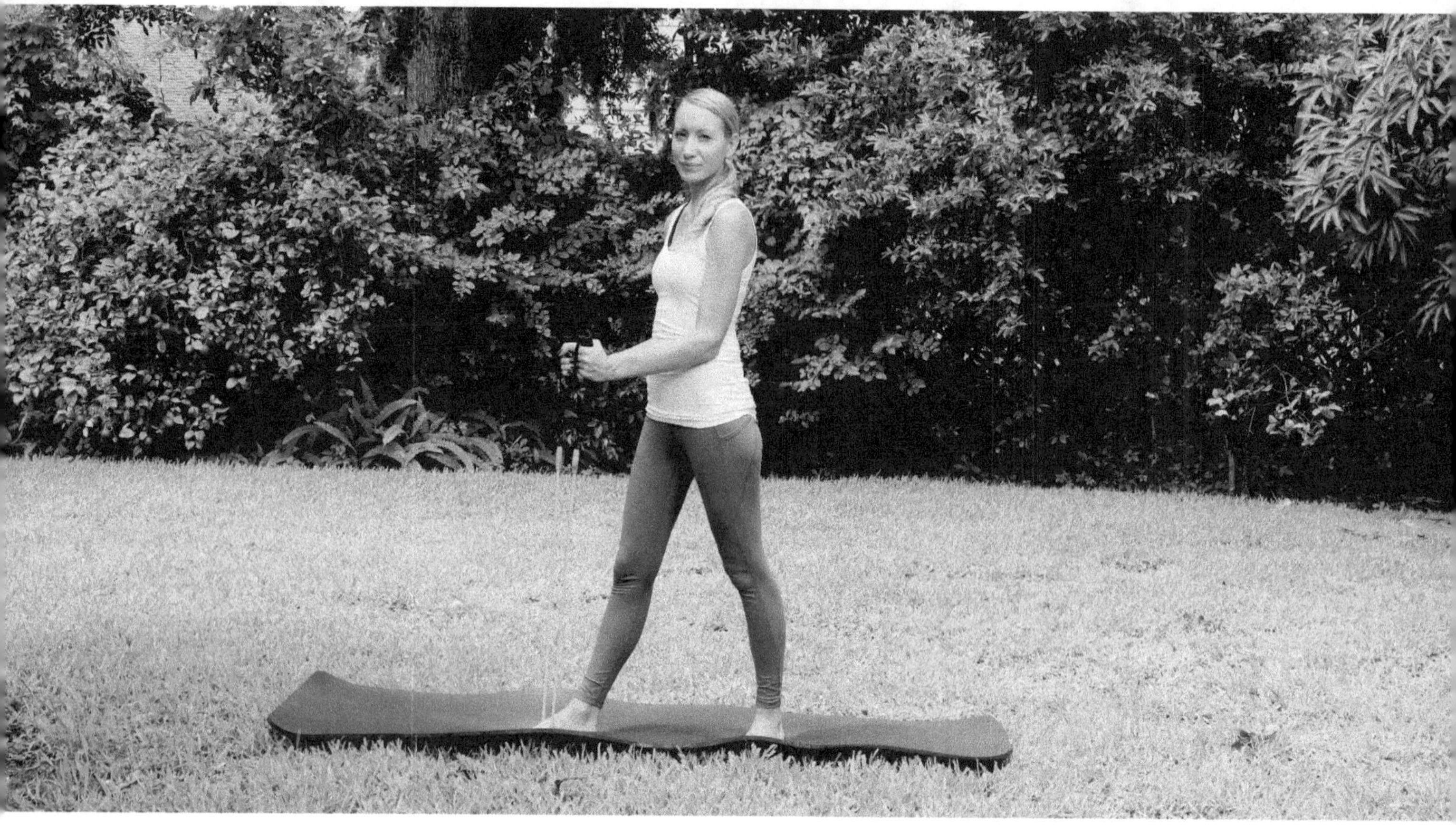

1. *Stand in a staggered stance and place cable under your back foot with knees slightly bent.*

2. *Grasp handles and position your arms at your sides.*

3. *Raise your arms up and inward in front of your chest with your arms slightly bent and your palms facing inwards.*

4. *Return to start and repeat.*

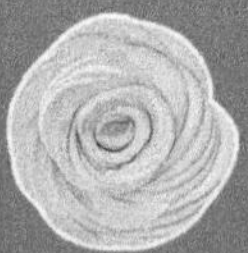

How to do Arm Curls

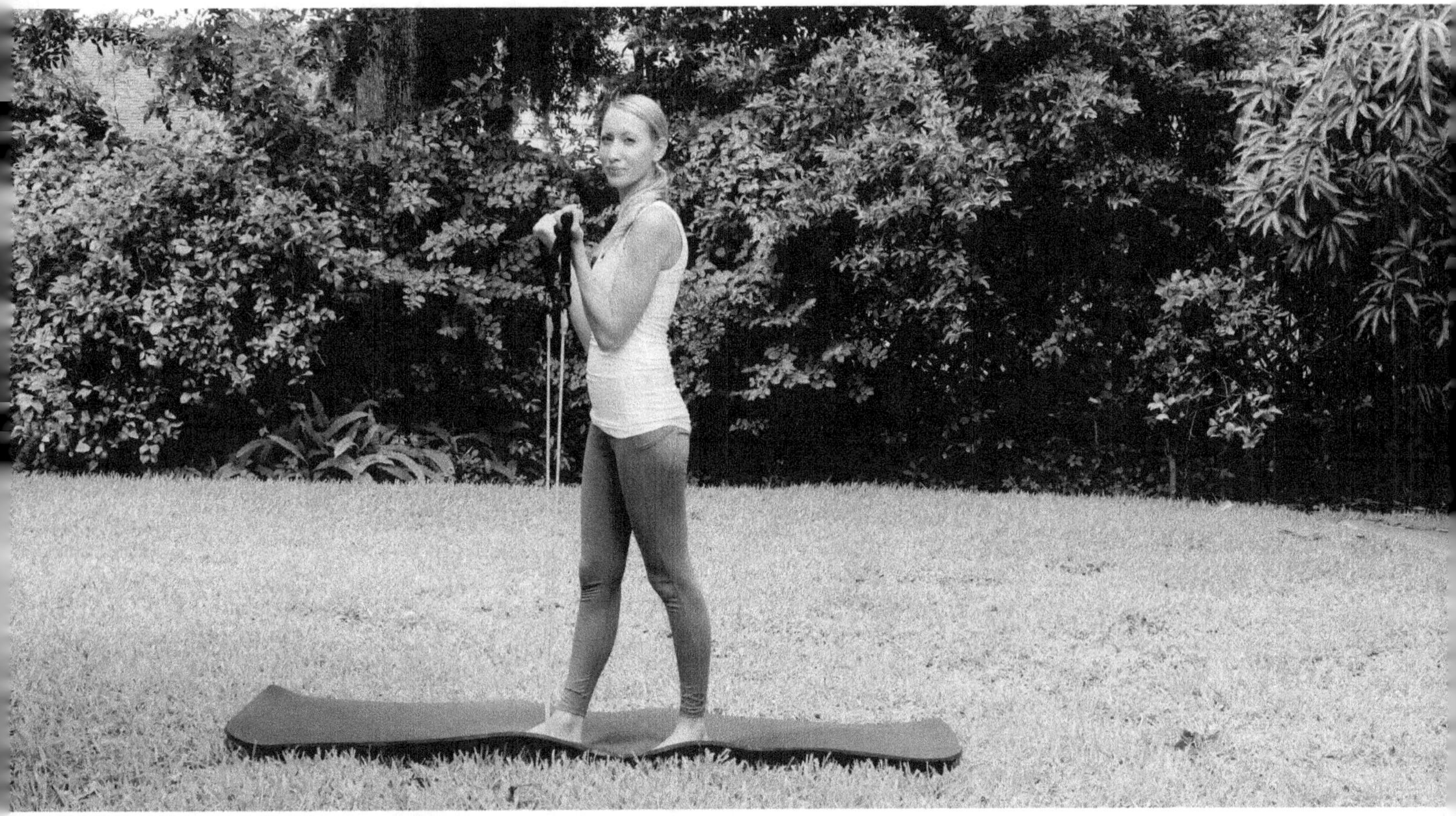

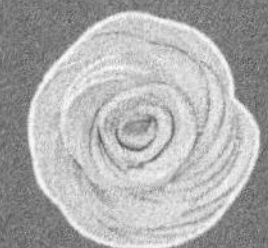

1. *Stand in a staggered stance and place cable under your front foot with knees slightly bent.*

2. *Grab handles and position your arms at your sides.*

3. *Bend your arms and bring your hands in front of you to shoulder height.*

4. *Keep your wrists firm and elbows at your sides.*

5. *Return to start and repeat.*

How to do Side Raises

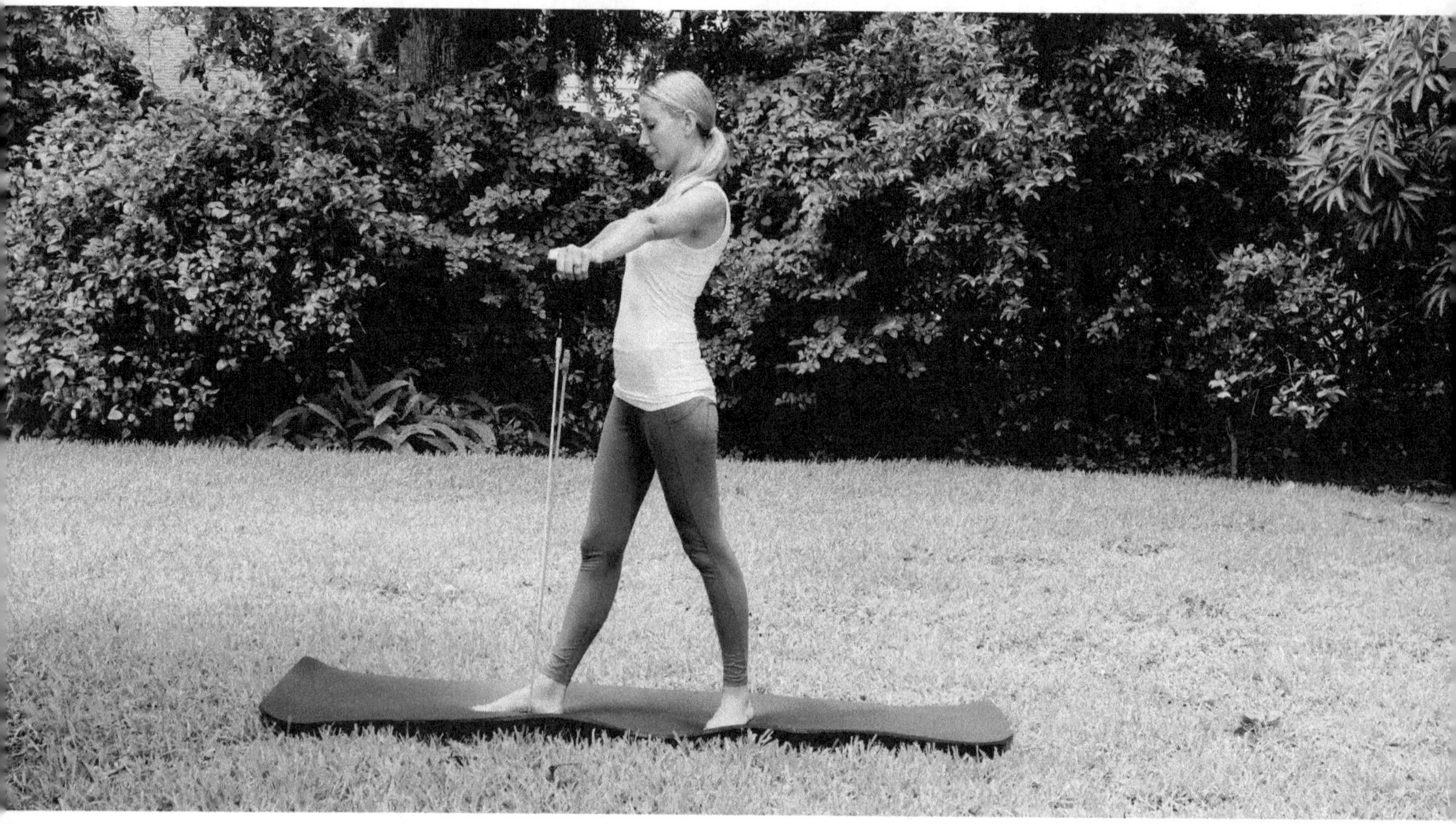

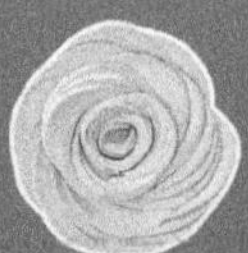

1. *Stand in a staggered stance and place the cable under your front foot with your knees slightly bent.*

2. *Grasp handles with palms facing your thighs and position your arms at your sides directly under your shoulders.*

3. *Lift your arms up and away from your sides to your shoulder height.*

4. *Keep your wrists firm and elbows soft.*

5. *Return to start and repeat.*

How to do Arm Extensions

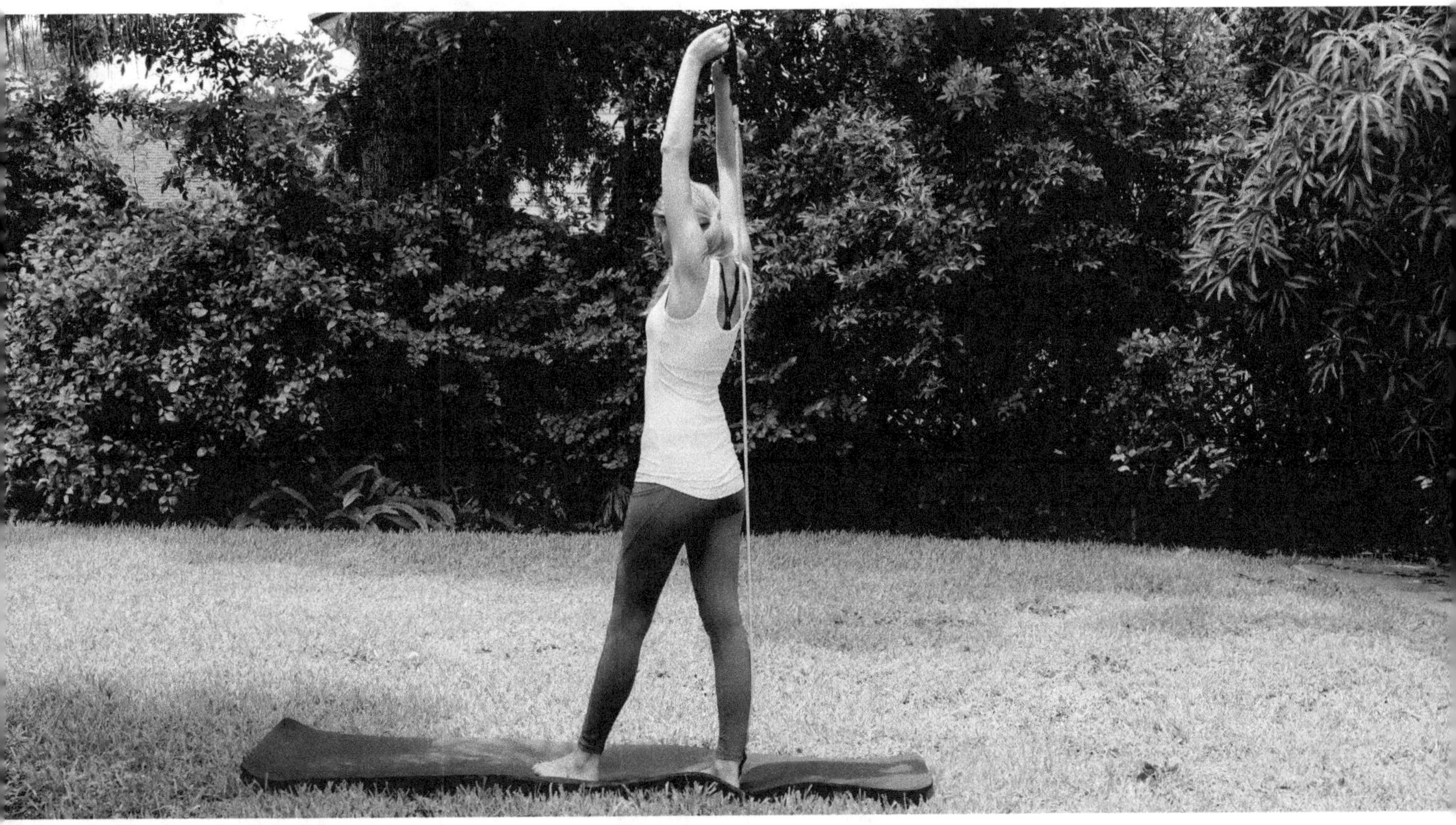

1. Stand in a staggered stance and place your back foot onto the cable with your knees slightly bent.

2. Grasp one handle with both hands, bend your arms and position them behind your head.

3. Straighten your arms overhead directly above your shoulders.

4. Keep your wrists firm and your upper arms stationary.

5. Return to start and repeat.

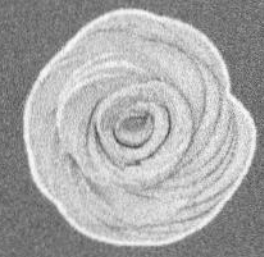

Resistance Loop Band Workouts

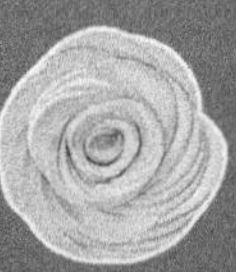

How to do Leg Extensions

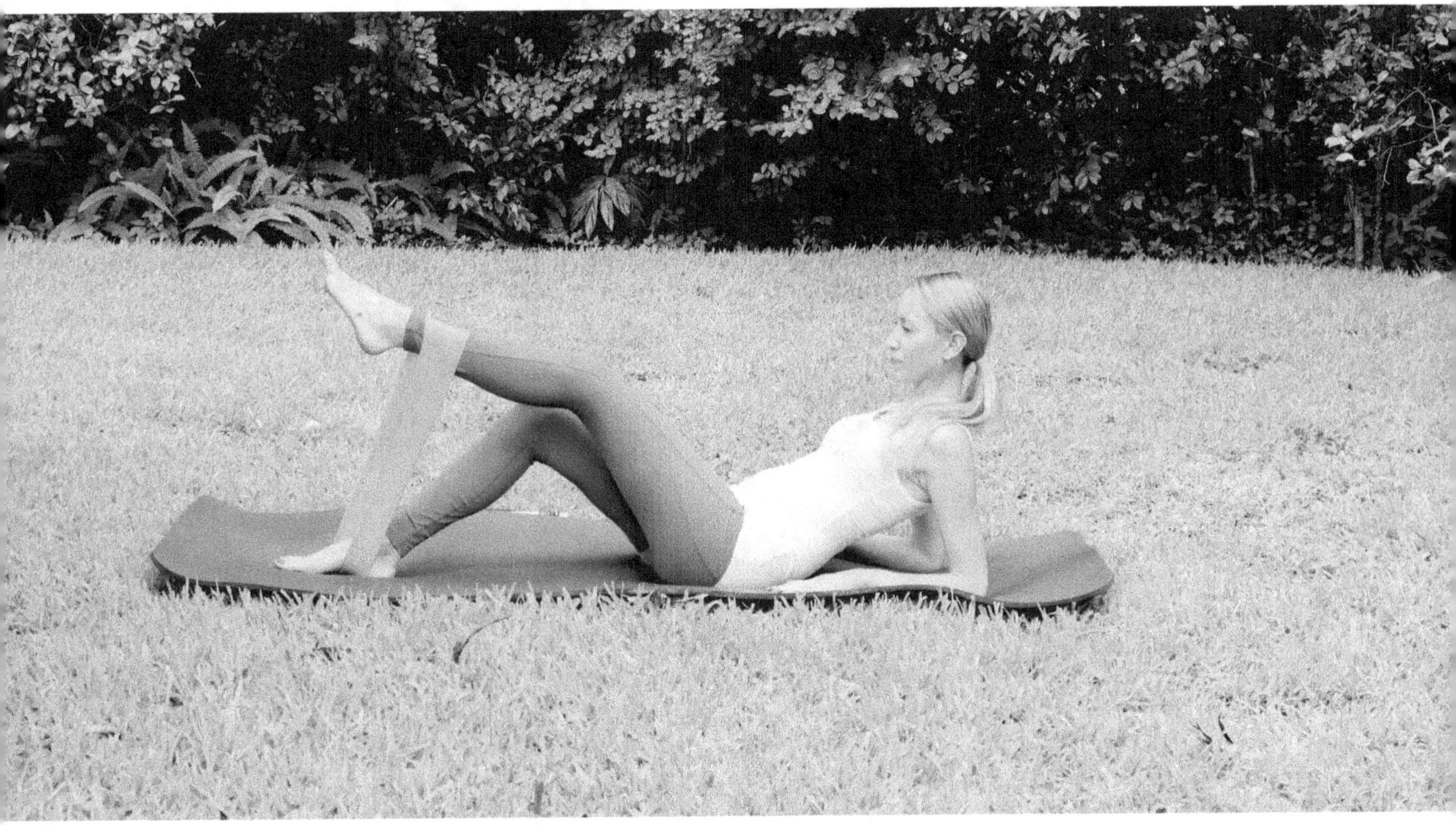

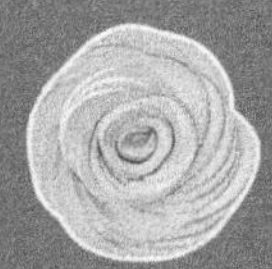

1. *Sit on the floor, bend your legs and secure your right foot on one end of the loop while the other end of the loop is around your left ankle.*

2. *Lie back and support your upper body with your forearms.*

3. *Straighten your left leg with the loop around your left ankle, whilst your right foot is stationary.*

4. *Return to the start and repeat. Alternate sides left and right sides.*

How to do Side Steps

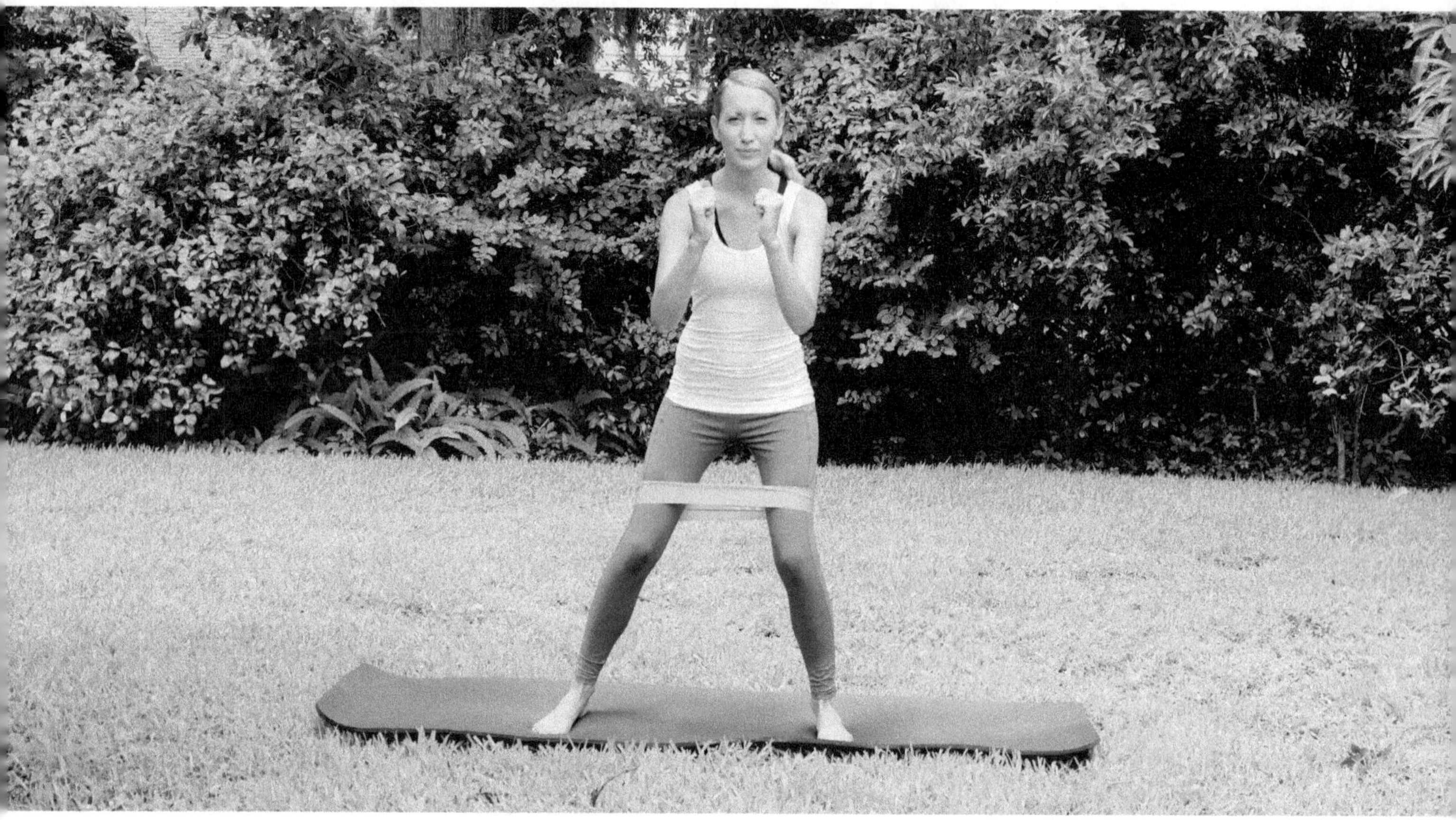

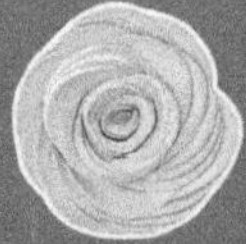

1. *Whilst in a standing position, secure the loop of the band above your knees being hip-width apart and knees slightly bent.*

2. *Keep your arms at your sides, your head up, and hips square.*

3. *Keep one leg stationary with your foot on the floor, while stepping out sideways with your other leg, stretching the loop.*

4. *Keep knees bent, hips down and shoulders square.*

5. *Return to start and repeat. Alternate left and right sides.*

How to do Kick Backs

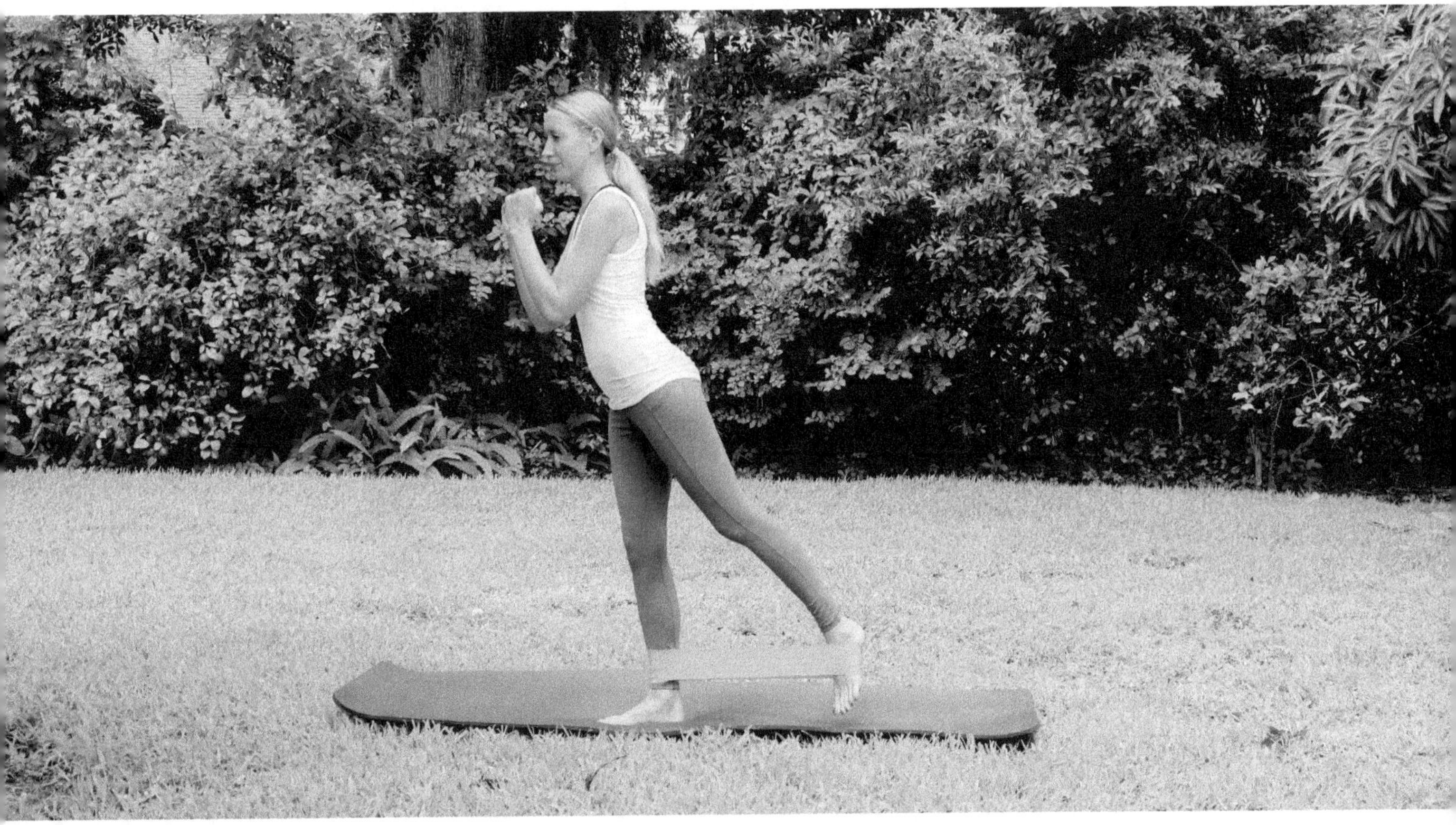

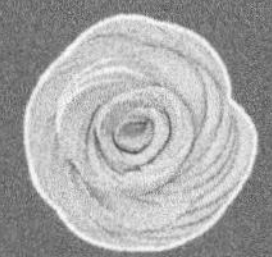

1. Place loop of the band just above ankle of non-exercise leg and around the other foot you will exercise.

2. Stand and balance on the leg you are not exercising, and bend the other leg behind you with your foot slightly off the floor.

3. Straighten and lift bent leg backwards, keeping toes pointed towards the floor.

4. Keep hips and shoulders square.

5. Return to start and repeat, then alternate sides.

How to do Outer Leg Lifts

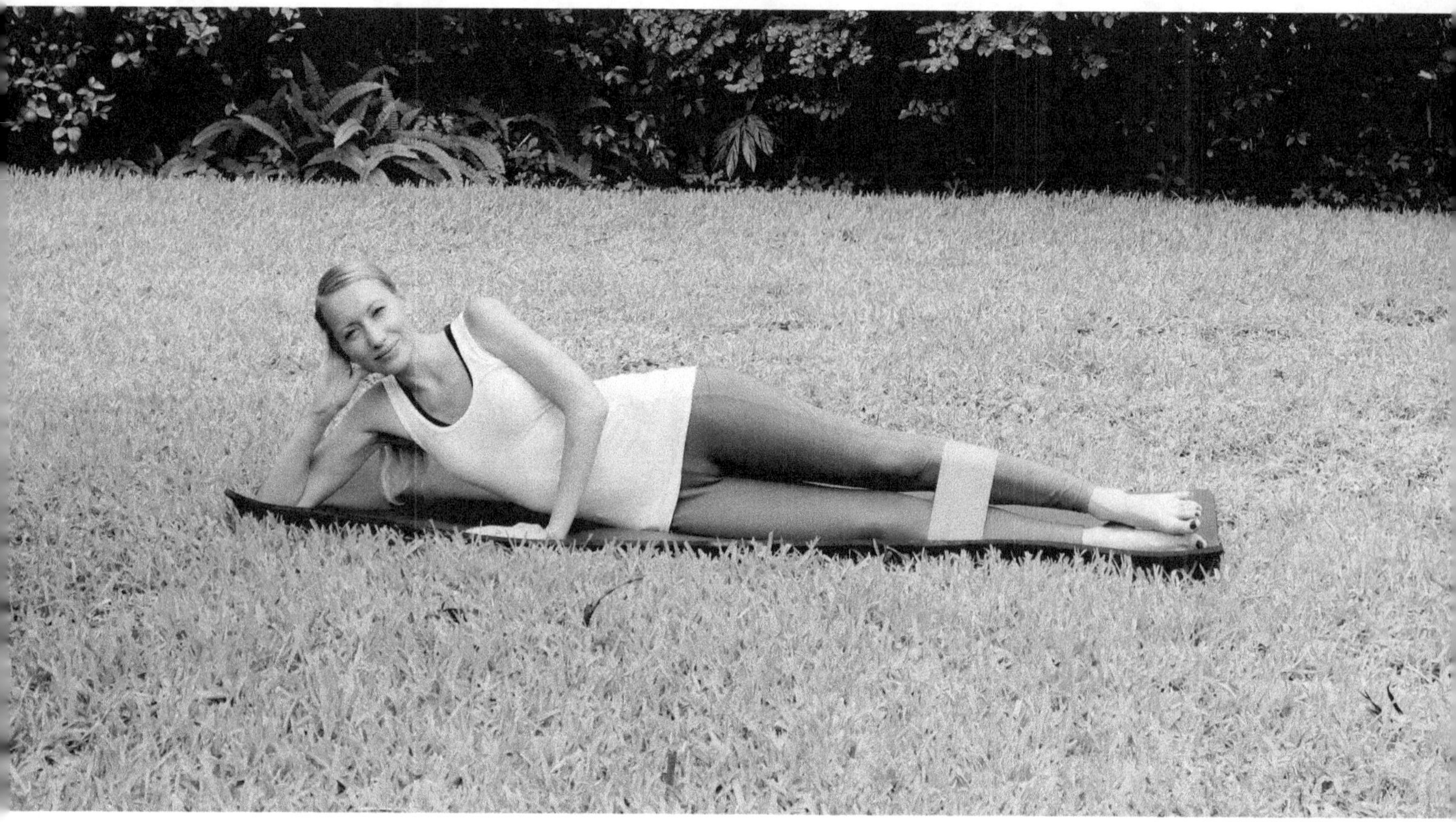

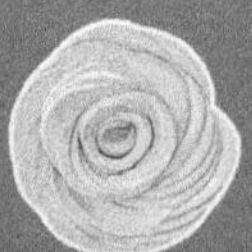

1. Secure the loop of the band around both legs, just below the knees and straighten legs.

2. Lie down on one side of your hip, with your bottom arm bent, your head supported in your hand, your top arm bent and your hand positioned flat on the floor in front of you.

3. Lift your top leg straight up and away from your bottom leg which should stay stationary on the floor.

4. Return to start and repeat, then alternate sides.

How to do Inner Leg Lift

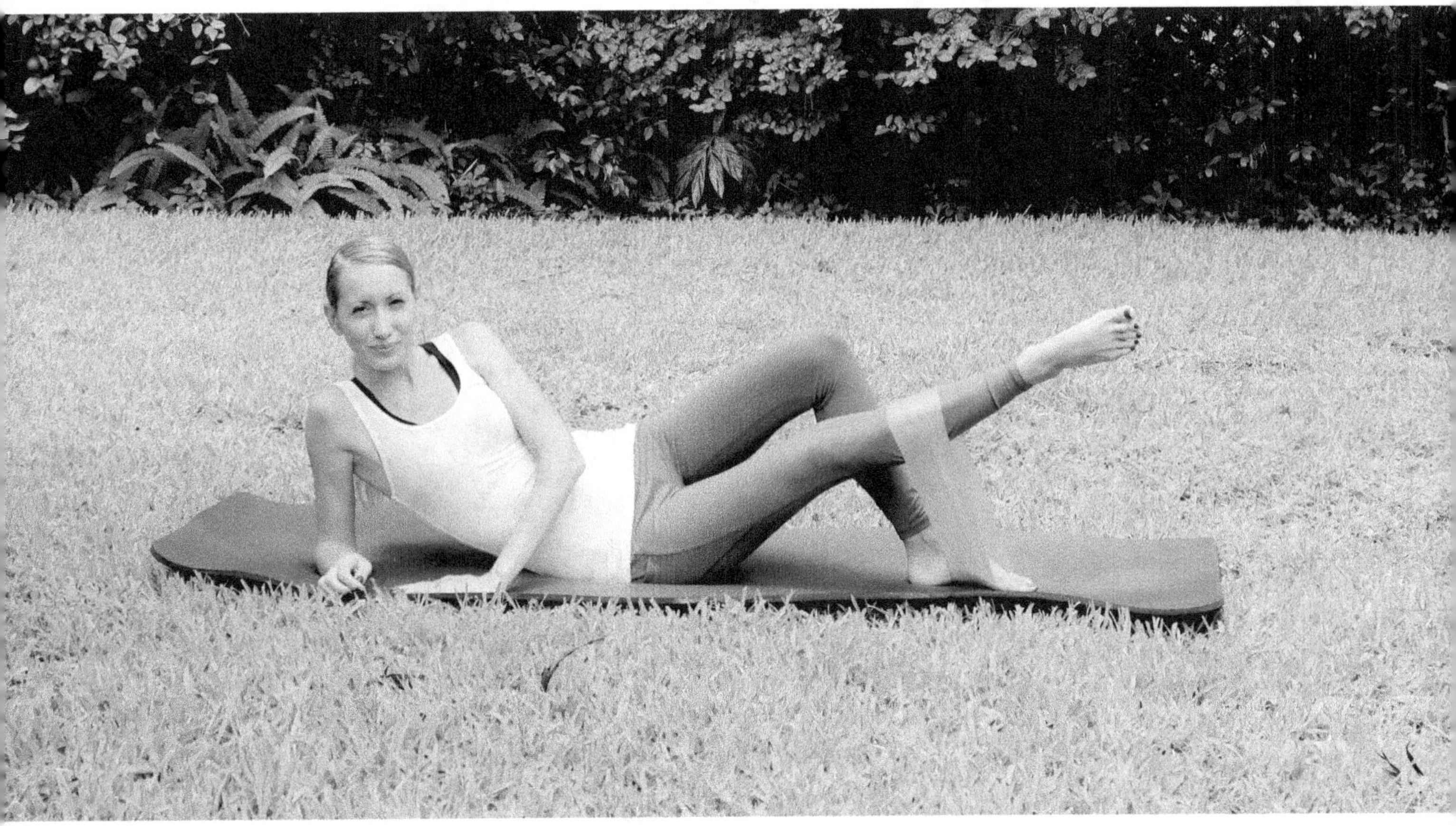

1. Lie on your side and secure the loop around your foot and around your shin.

2. Bend the leg with the loop around your foot, so that your foot is flat on the floor and then straighten your other leg with loop around your shin.

3. Bend your arms and position your bottom elbow directly below your shoulder and place your upper arms hand on the floor in front of your hip.

4. Return to start and repeat, then alternate sides.

How to do Leg Curls

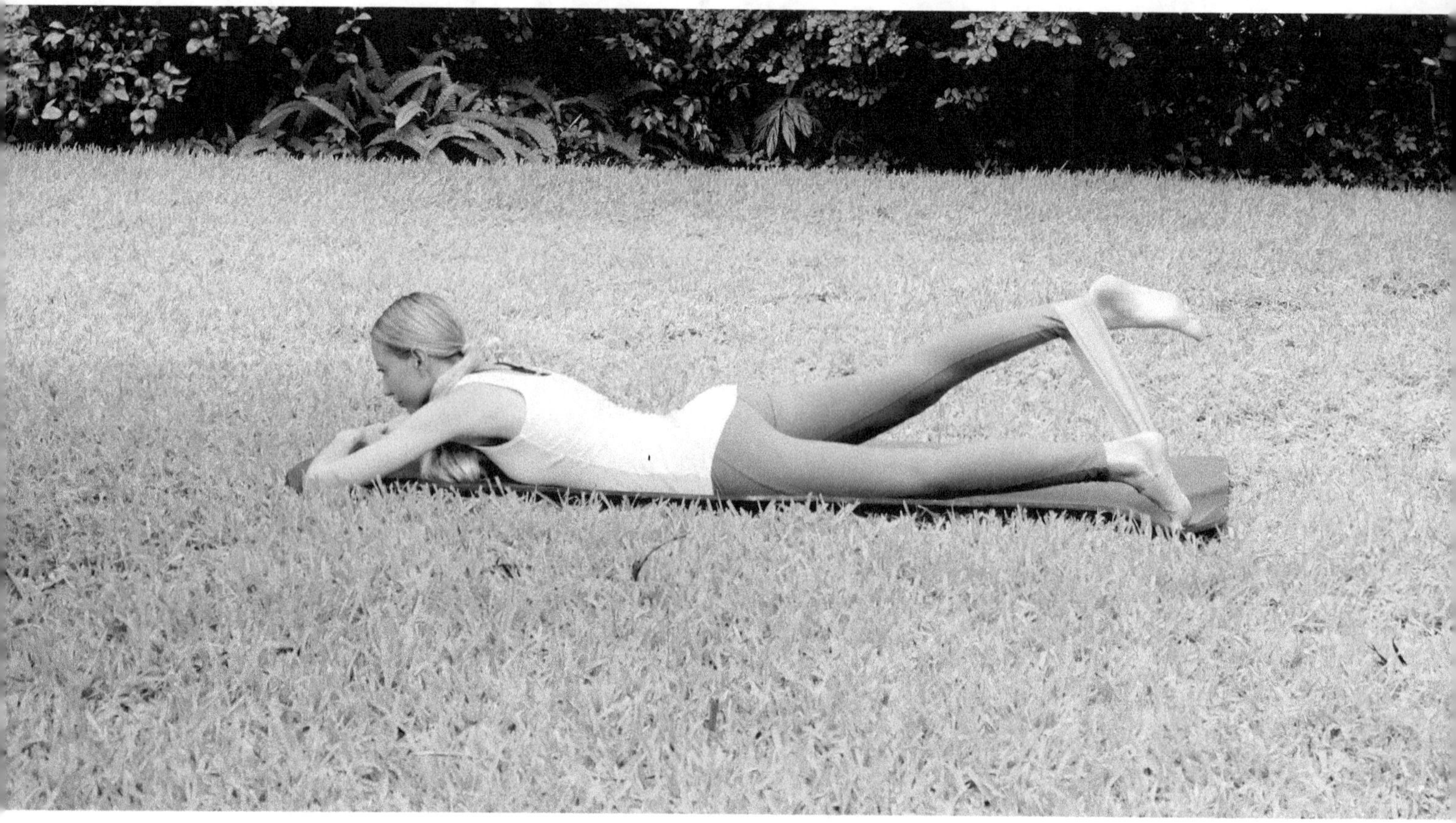

1. Place the band around your one foot and around your other legs ankle.

2. Lie on your stomach with your legs straight and feet hip-width apart.

3. Bend your arms, rest your head on your hands, and press hips into the floor.

4. Bend the leg with the band around your ankle towards your buttocks whilst keeping the other legs toes firmly on the ground.

5. Return to start and repeat, then alternate sides.

www.ketoveo.com

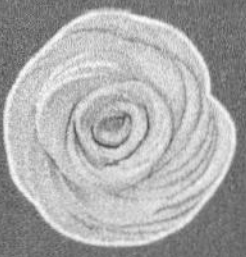

How to do Ankle Jumping Jacks

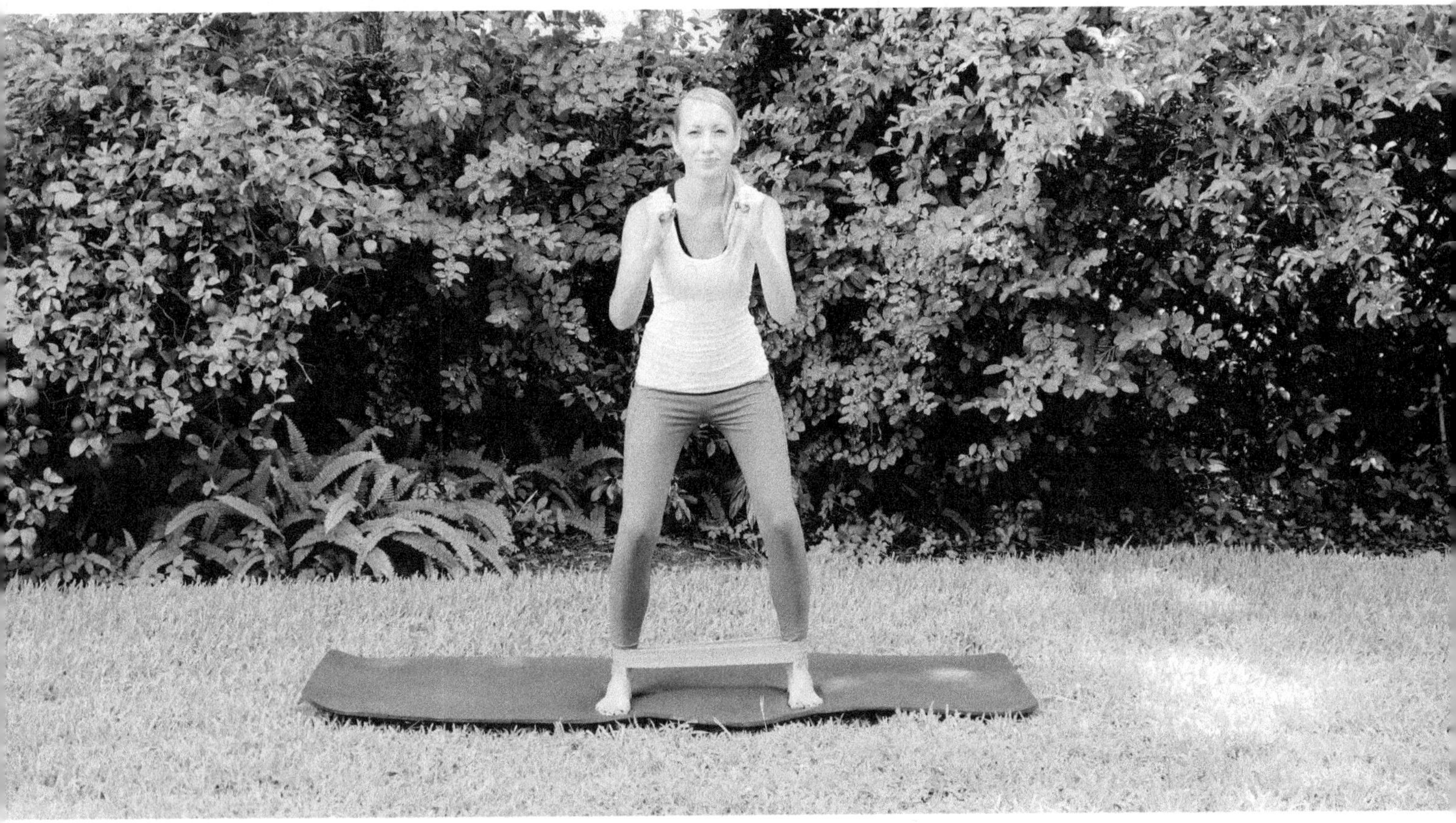

1. Place the band around your ankles.

2. Stand in a quarter-squat position (a shallower squat), with your feet about hip-width apart, hands at your chest.

3. Jump your feet out and in for 1 rep. Try not to let your body pop up too high, and land with your weight mostly in your heels, not your toes

4. Do 20 reps.

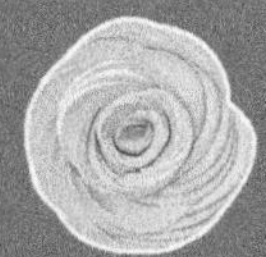

How to do Lateral Band Walks

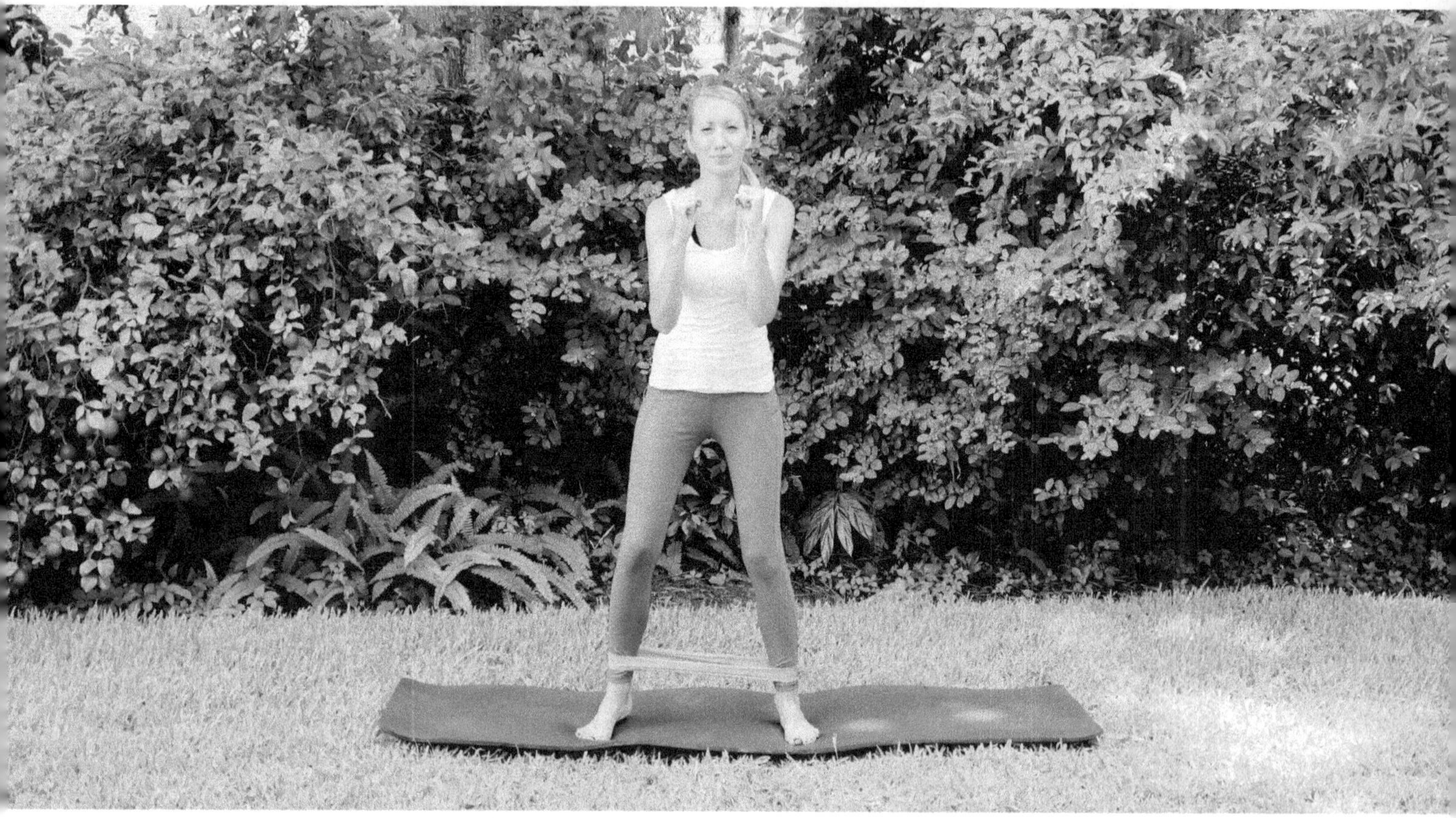

1. *Place the band around your ankles.*

2. *Stand in a quarter-squat position (a shallower squat), with your feet about hip-width apart, hands at your chest or on your hips.*

3. *Take a step to the right with your right foot, so that your feet are shoulder-width apart. Then, follow with your left so that your feet are hip-width apart again.*

4. *Take three steps to the right, and then three back to the left. That's 1 rep. Try to keep your weight in the center, keep your core engaged, and keep constant tension in the band.*

5. *Do 20 reps.*

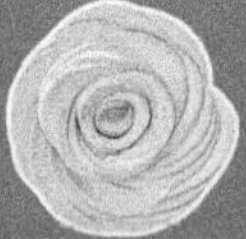

How to do Standing Glute Kickbacks

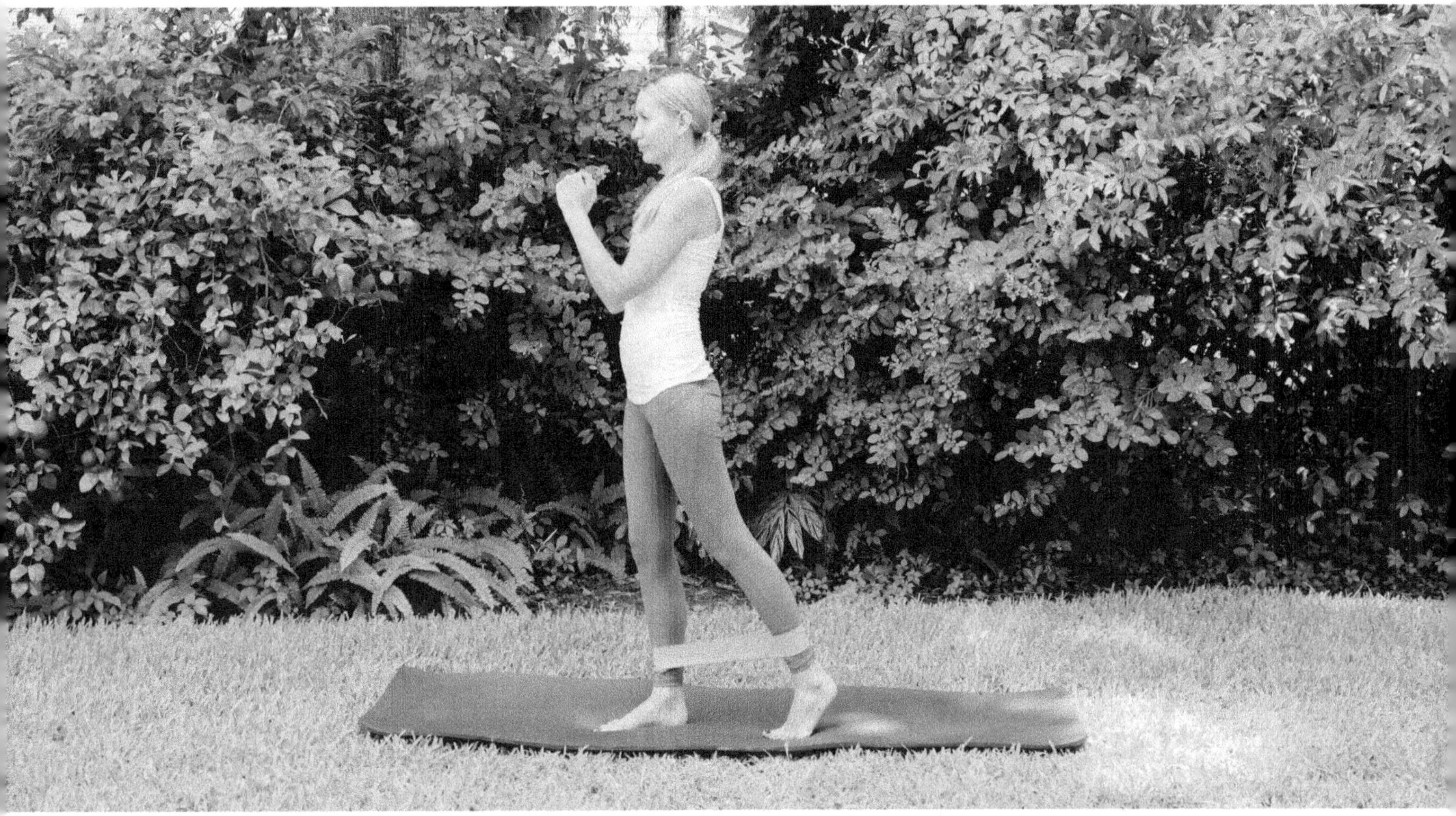

1. Place the band around your ankles.

2. With your hands at your chest or on your hips, shift all your weight into your right leg and place your left toes on the ground about an inch diagonally behind your right heel, so there is tension in the band.

3. Squeeze your abs and tuck your pelvis under as you kick your left leg back about 6 inches. Keep the knee straight.

4. Return your left foot to the ground, keeping tension in the band, for 1 rep. If you feel your lower back arching when you kick, make the movement smaller. Try not to put any weight on the leg that's kicking as it comes back down to the ground.

5. Do 20 reps. Switch sides and repeat.

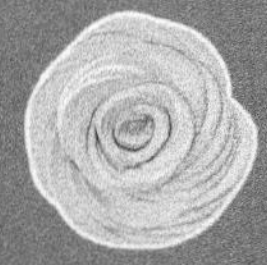

How to do Banded Walks

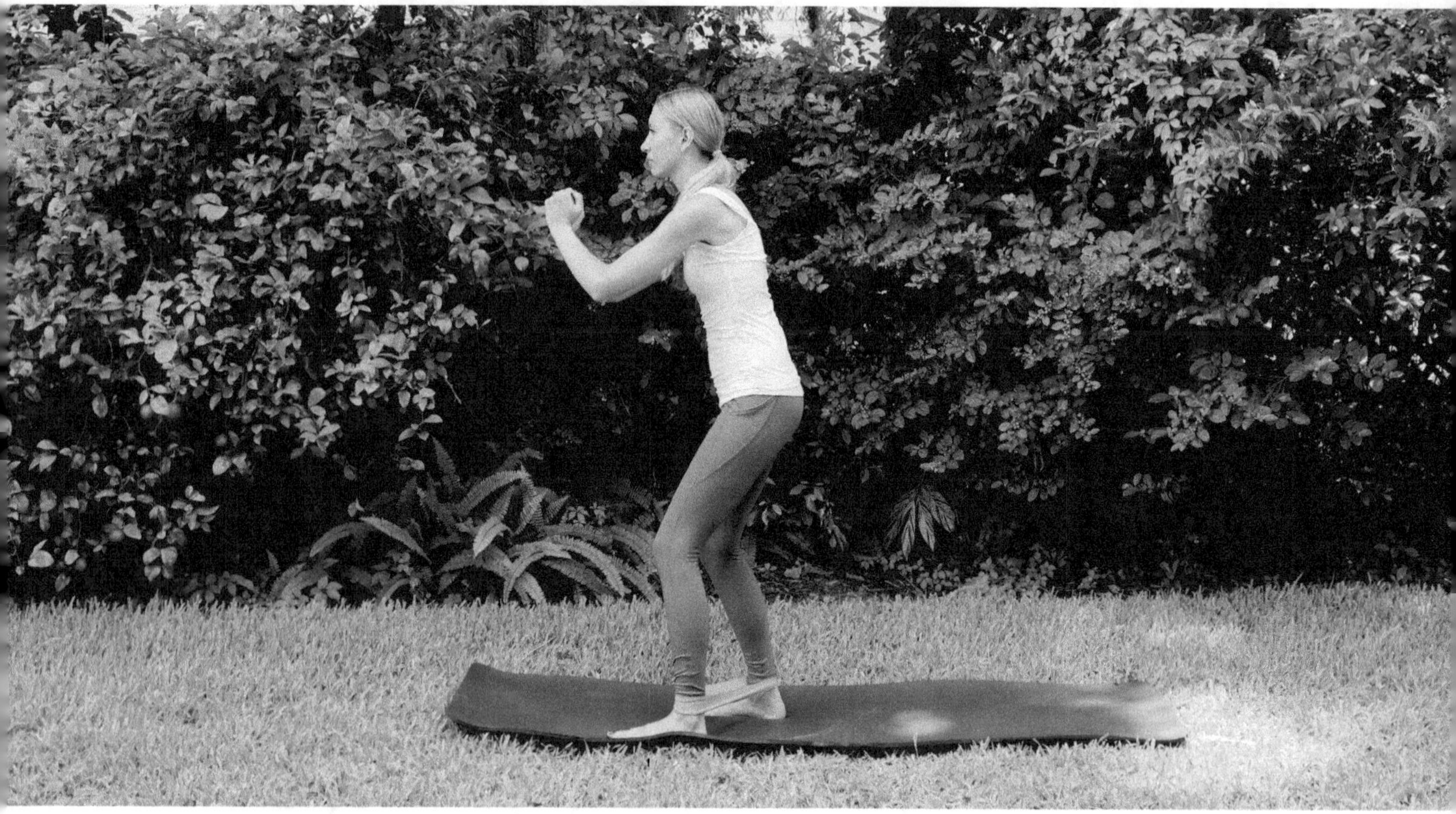

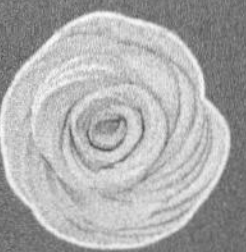

1. Place the band around your ankles.

2. Stand with your feet hip-width apart. Bend your knees a few inches and hinge forward at the hips, keeping your abs engaged and glutes tight.

3. Take 10 steps forward.

4. Take 10 steps backward. That's 20 reps. Be sure to keep your back flat and shoulders back so you're not hunching over.

How to do Squat to Lateral Leg Lifts

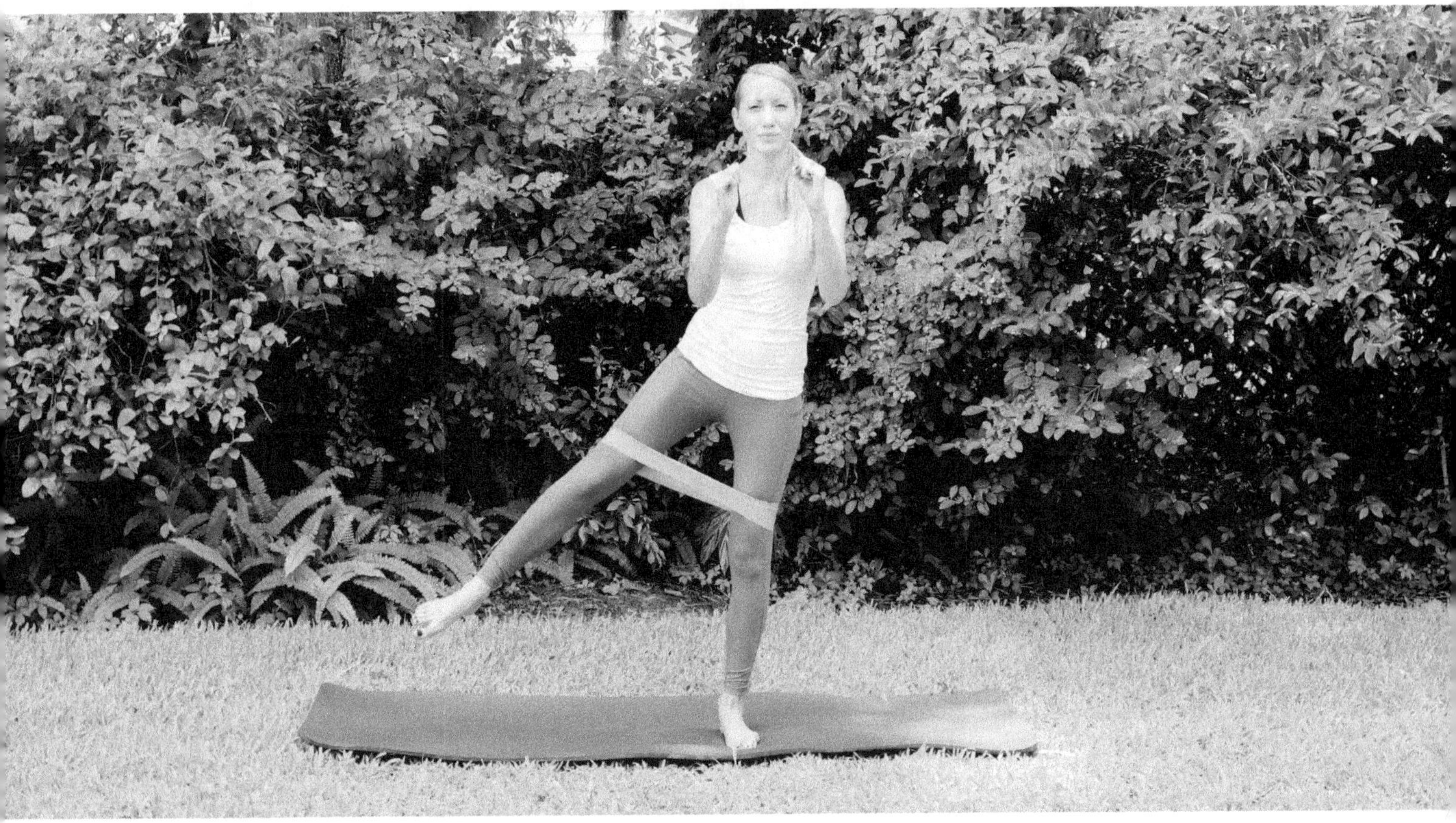

1. Place the band just above your knees.

2. Stand with your feet hip-width apart, with your hands at your chest or on your hips.

3. Bend your knees and push your butt back to lower into a squat.

4. Stand back up and lift your right leg out to the side, keeping your knee straight.

5. Return your right leg to the floor.

6. Squat again. This time when you stand back up, lift your left leg out to the side, keeping your knee straight. Make sure your chest is lifted and that you're not rounding or arching your back.

7. Return your left leg to floor. That's 1 rep.

8. Do 20 reps, alternating sides.

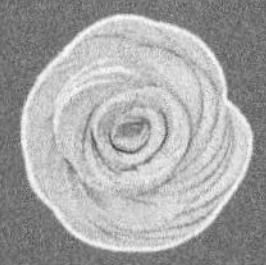

How to do Clamshells

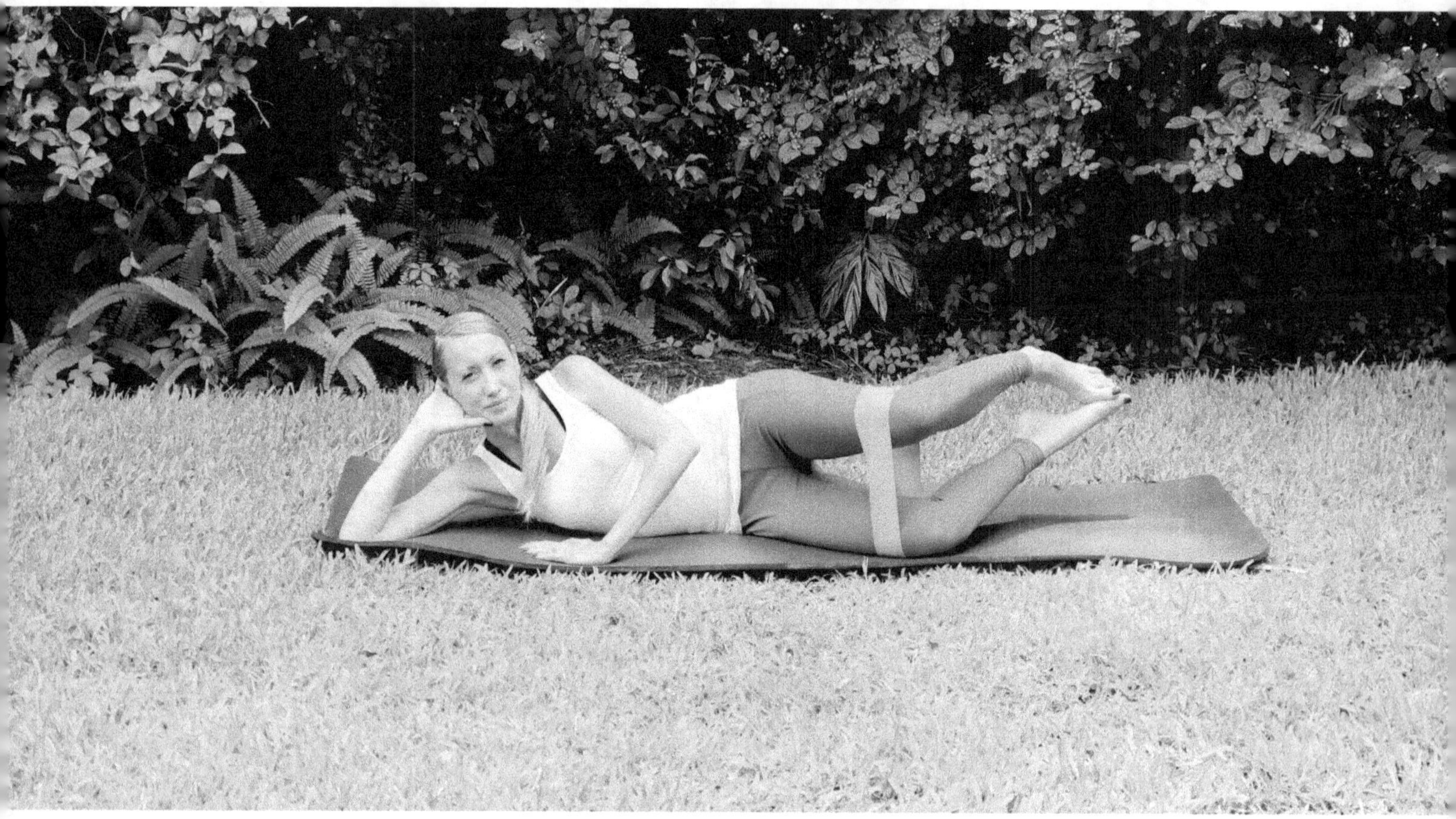

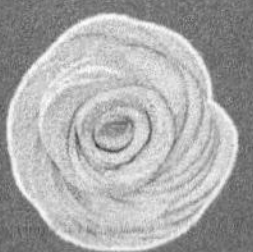

1. Place the band above your knees.

2. Lie on your side, with your head resting on your bottom hand. Elevate your feet to hip height (if you can), keeping your knees touching the floor.

3. Keep your feet together as you lift your top knee toward the ceiling.

4. Slowly lower the top knee down to hover right above the bottom knee. That's 1 rep. If it's too difficult to open up your knees with your feet in the air, leave them on the ground and do the same movement.

5. Do 20 reps. Switch sides and repeat.

How to do Hip Bride Pulses

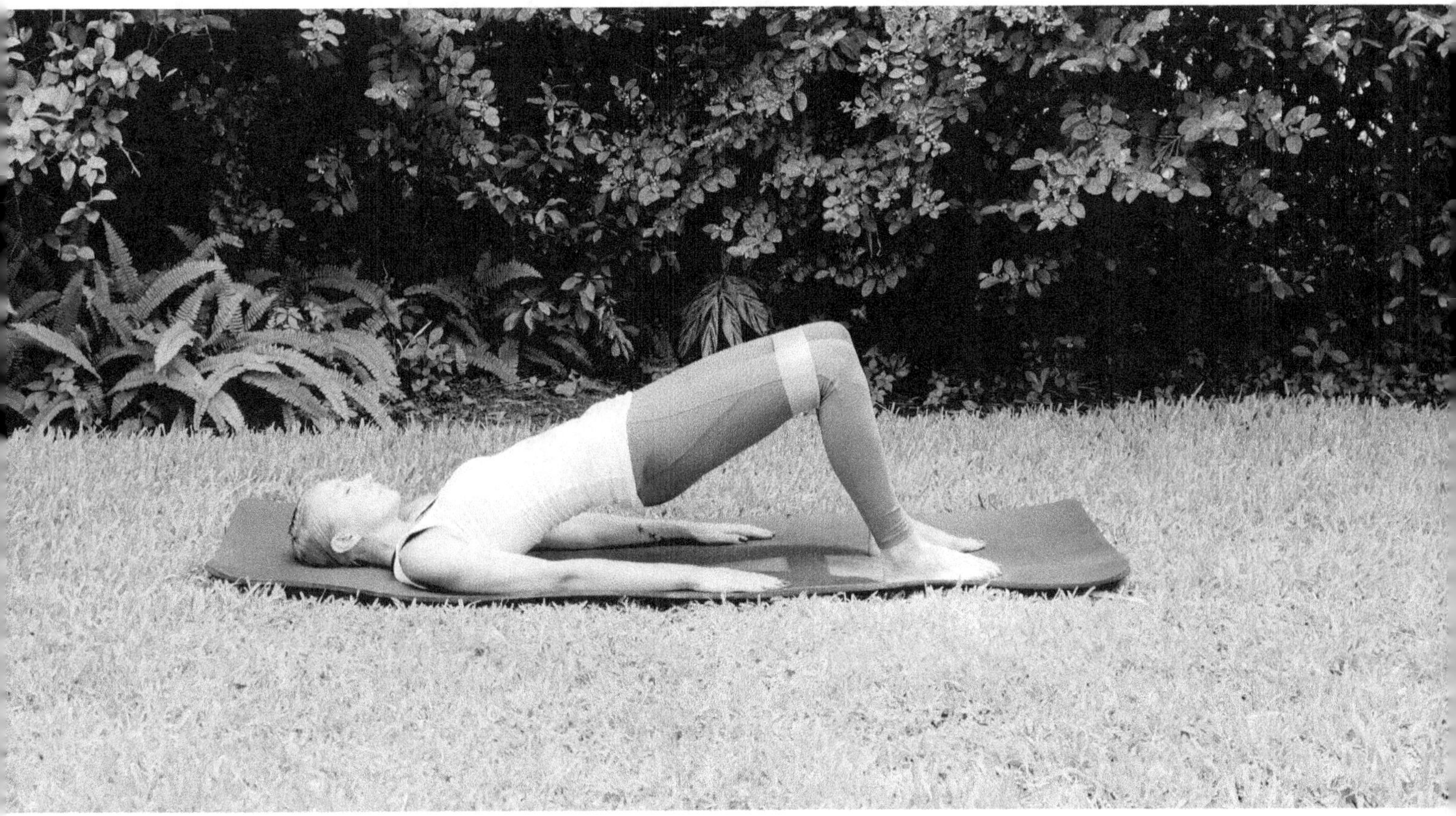

1. Place the band just above your knees.

2. Lie on your back with your hands at your sides, knees bent, and feet flat on floor hip-width apart.

3. Squeeze your glutes and abs and lift your hips a few inches off the floor. Walk your feet together.

4. Hold the bridge, and push your knees out to the sides, keeping your feet touching.

5. Slowly return your knees to touch for 1 rep. Keep your pelvis tucked under, with no arch in your back, and pull your belly button to your spine to maintain correct form.

6. Do 20 reps.

How to do Fire Hydrants

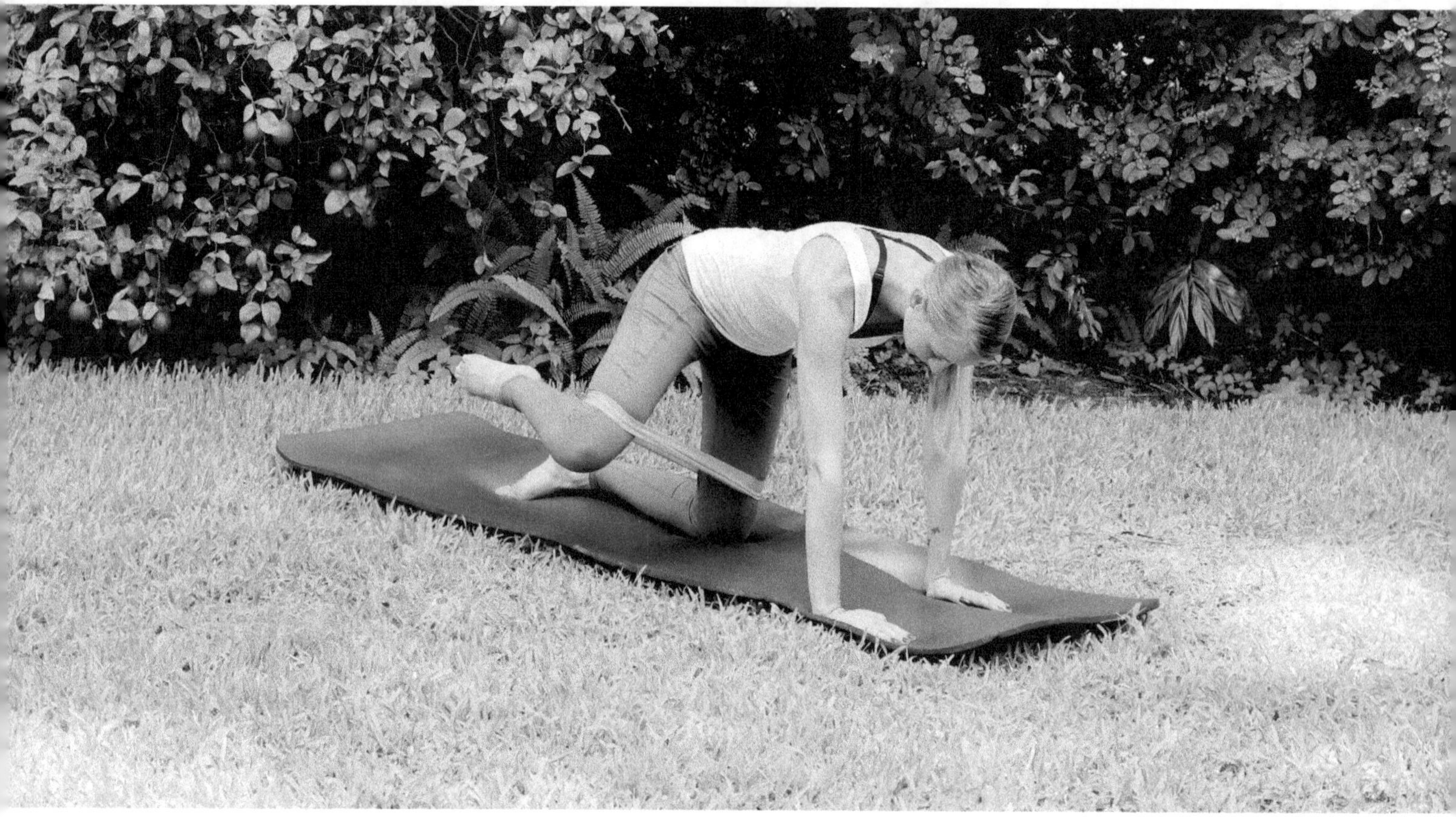

1. Place the band just above your knees.

2. Start on all fours with your hands under your shoulders and knees under your hips.

3. Without shifting your hips, left your left knee out to the side.

4. Slowly return to starting position for 1 rep. Keep your core engaged, so you're stabilized and not shifting your hips whilst keeping a constant resistance in the band.

5. Do 20 reps. Switch sides and repeat.

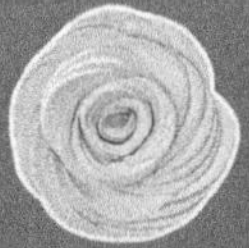

How to do Hip Bridges With Alternating Leg Extension

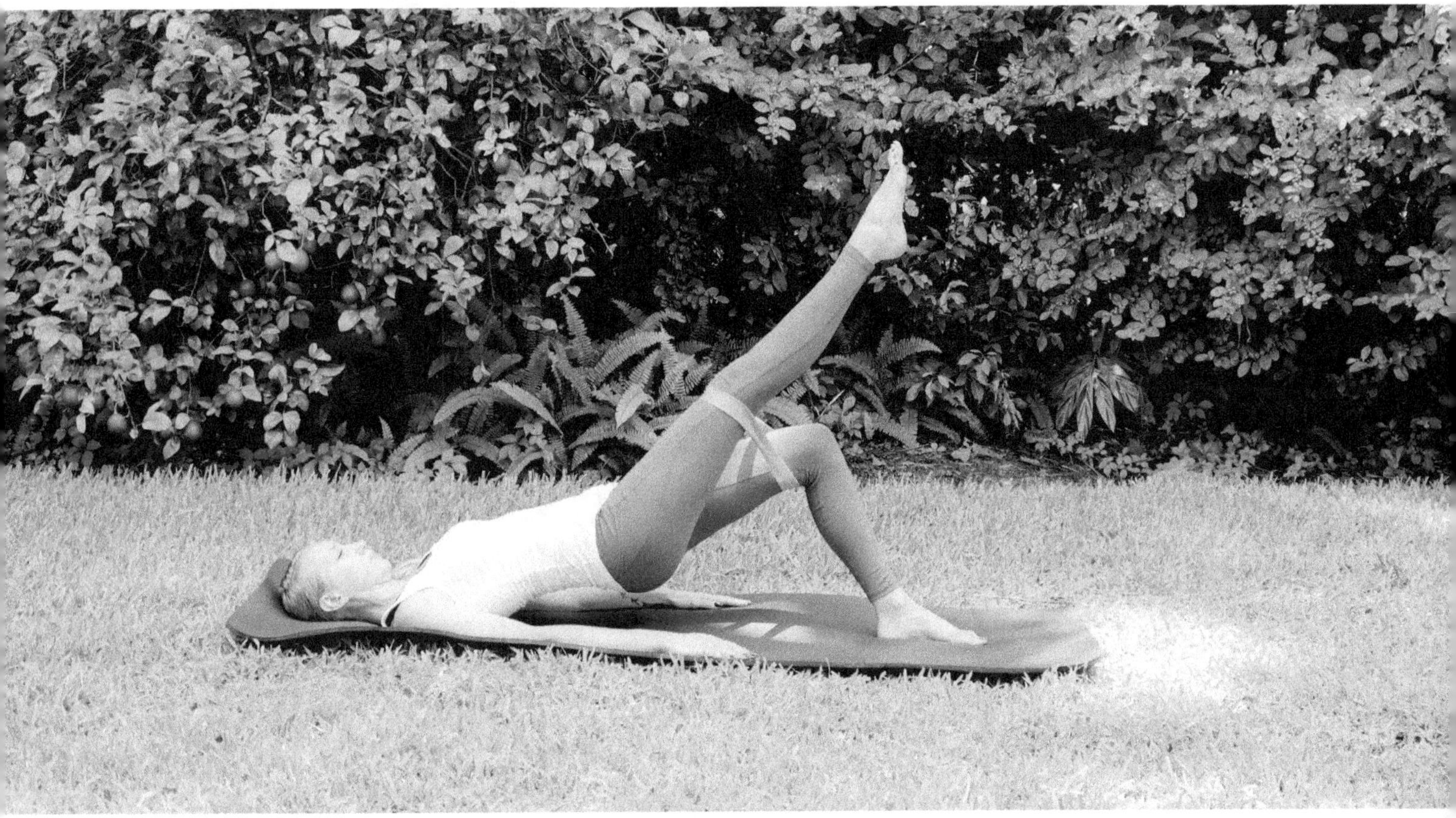

1. Place the band just above your knees.

2. Lie on your back with your hands at your sides, knees bent, and feet flat on floor hip-width apart.

3. Squeeze your glutes and abs and lift your hips a few inches off the floor.

4. Extend your right leg until it's straight, keeping your knees in line.

5. Return your right leg to starting position. Bring your hips back down to the floor.

6. Lift your hips up again. Then, extend your left leg until it's straight.

7. Return your left leg to starting position. Bring your hips back down to the floor. That's 1 rep. Focus on touching your heels on the floor each time, not your toes.

8. Continue, alternating sides for 20 reps.

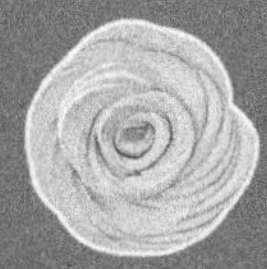

How to do Donkey Kicks

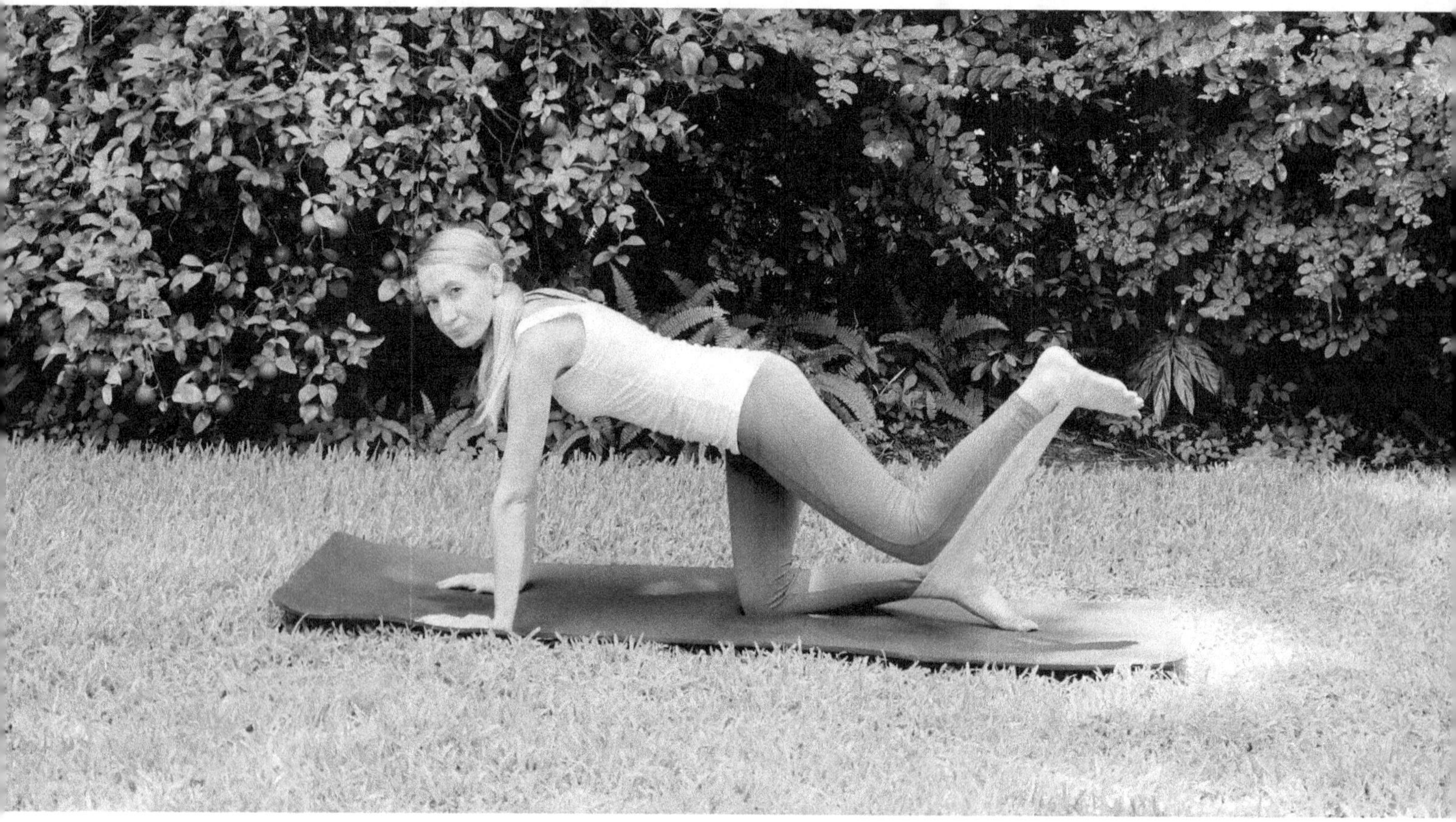

1. Loop the band around the bottom of your left foot and right ankle.

2. Start on all fours with your knees under your hips and hands under your shoulders.

3. Kick your left leg up, keeping your foot flexed and knees bent. Hold for 2 seconds at the top. The longer you hold the better the workout.

4. Return your left leg to floor for 1 rep.

5. Continue on the same side for 20 reps.

6. Switch sides and repeat.

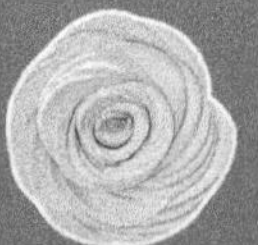

Basic Stretches Everyone Should Know

How to do Standing Hamstring Stretch

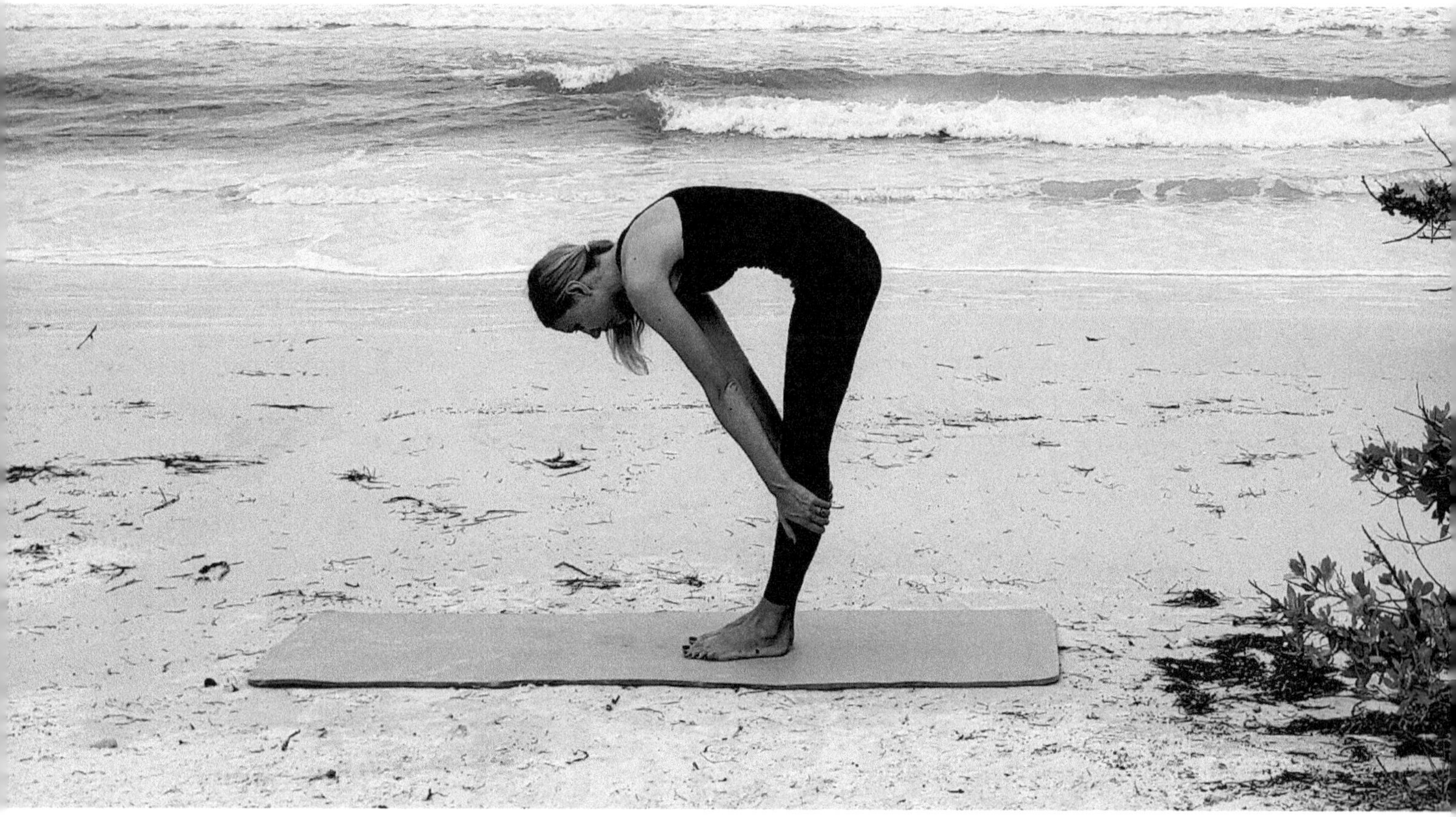

Hamstring Stretch - Stretches neck, back, glutes, hamstrings, calves

1. *Stand tall with your feet hip-width apart, knees slightly bent, arms by your sides.*

2. *Exhale as you bend forward at the hips, lowering your head toward floor, while keeping your head, neck and shoulders relaxed.*

3. *Wrap your arms around backs of your legs and hold anywhere from 45 seconds to two minutes.*

4. *Bend your knees and roll up when you're done.*

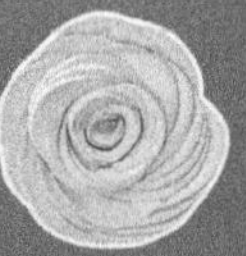

How to do Piriformis Stretch

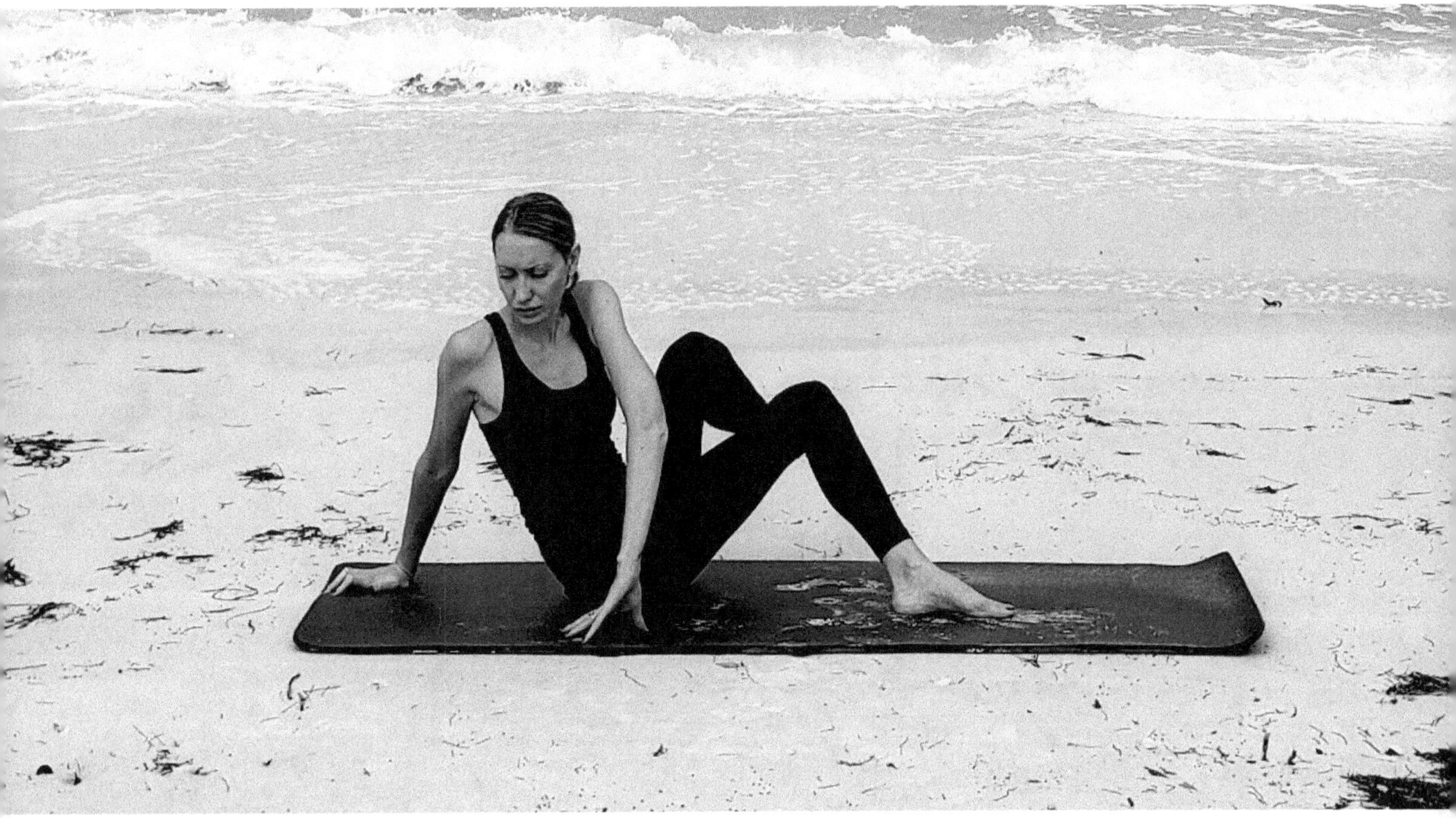

Piriformis Stretch - Stretches hips, back, glutes

1. *Sit on the floor with both legs extended in front of you.*

2. *Cross your right leg over your left, and place your right foot flat on the floor.*

3. *Place your right hand on the floor behind your body.*

4. *Place your left hand on your right quad or your left elbow on your right knee and press your right leg to the left as you twist your torso to the right, then repeat on the other side.*

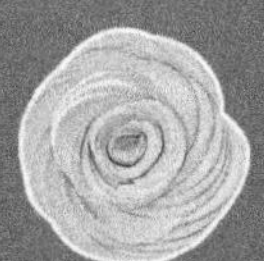

How to do Lunge With Spinal Twist

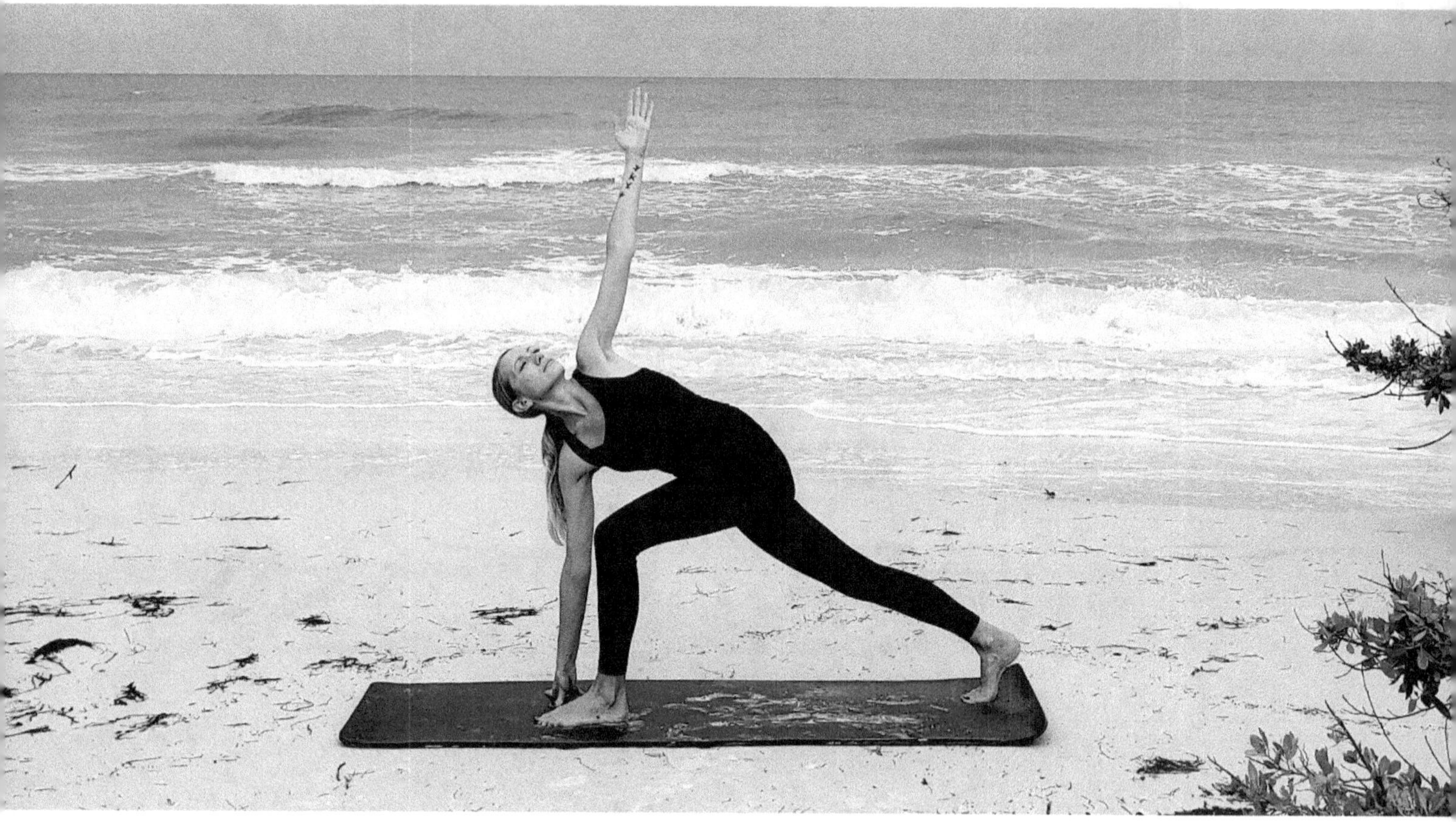

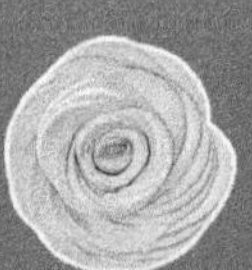

Lunge With Spinal Twist - Stretches hip flexors, quads, back

1. *Start standing with your feet together.*

2. *Take a big step forward with your left foot, so that you are in a staggered stance.*

3. *Bend your left knee and drop into a lunge, keeping your right leg straight behind you with your toes on the ground, so you feel a stretch at the front of your right thigh.*

4. *Place your right hand on the floor and twist your upper body to the left as you extend your left arm toward the ceiling.*

5. *Hold for 30 seconds to 2 minutes.*

6. *Repeat on the other side.*

www.ketoveo.com

How to do Triceps Stretch

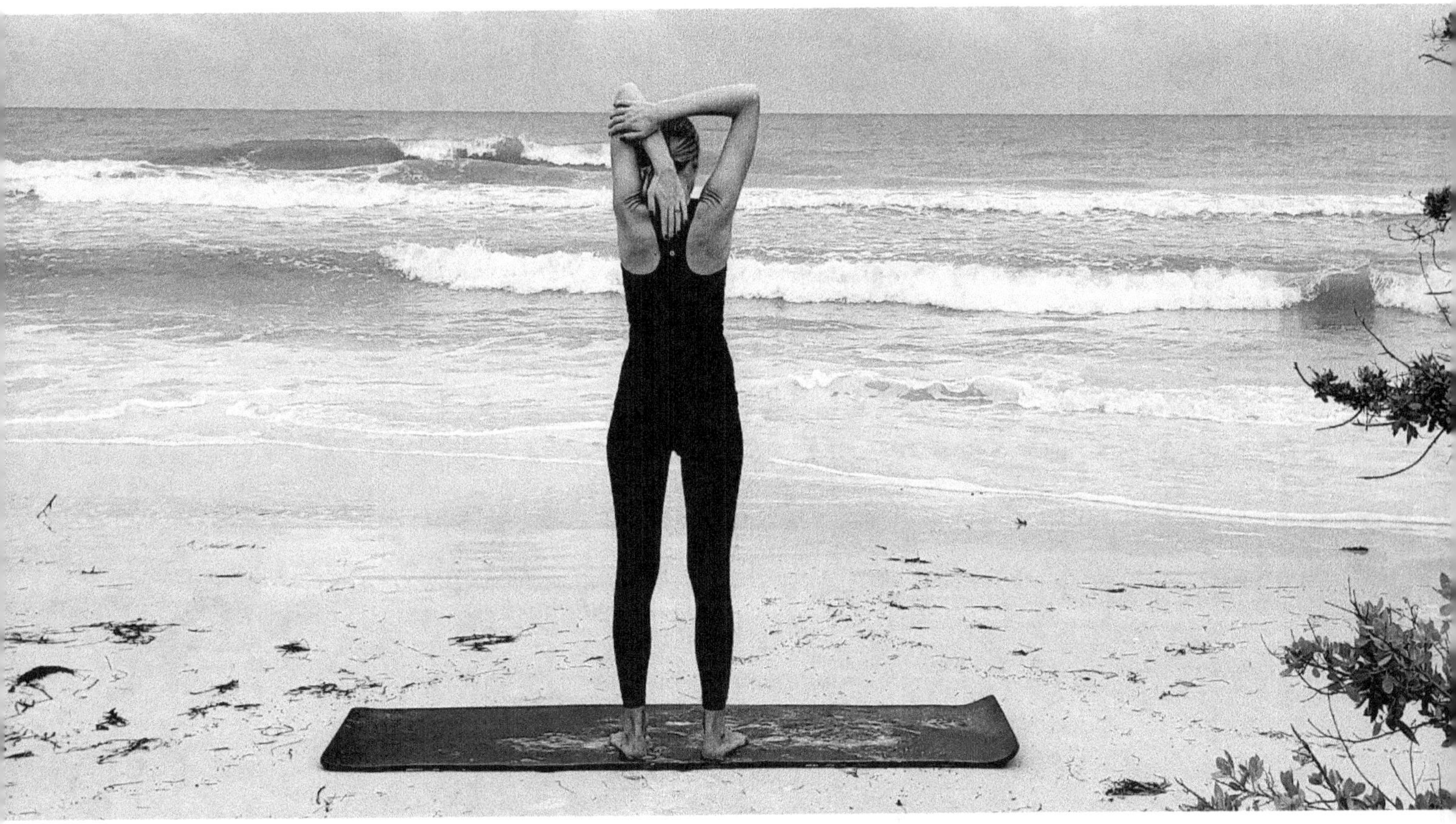

Triceps Stretch - Stretches neck, shoulders, back, triceps

1. *Kneel, sit, or stand tall with feet hip-width apart, arms extended overhead.*

2. *Bend your right elbow and reach your right hand to touch the top middle of your back.*

3. *Reach your left hand overhead and grasp just below your right elbow.*

4. *Gently pull your right elbow down and toward your head.*

5. *Switch arms and repeat.*

How to do Figure Four Stretch

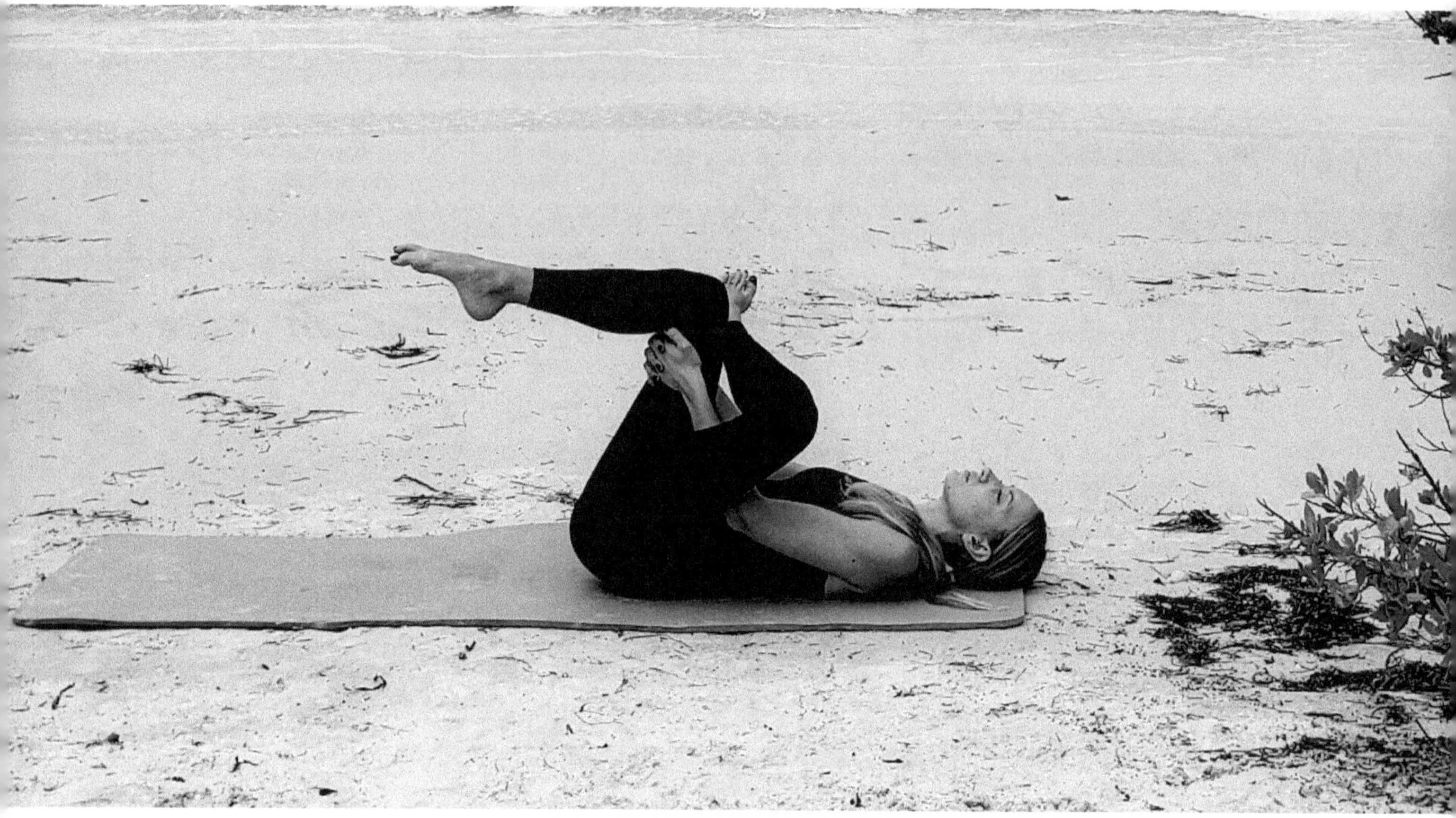

Figure Four Stretch - Stretches hips, glutes, lower back, hamstrings

1. Lie on your back with your feet flat on the floor.

2. Cross your left foot over your right quad.

3. Lift your right leg off the floor. Grab onto the back of your right leg and gently pull it toward your chest.

4. When you feel a comfortable stretch, hold there. Hold for 30 seconds to 2 minutes.

5. Switch sides and repeat.

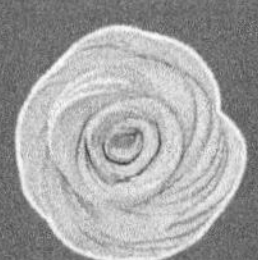

How to do 90/90 Stretch

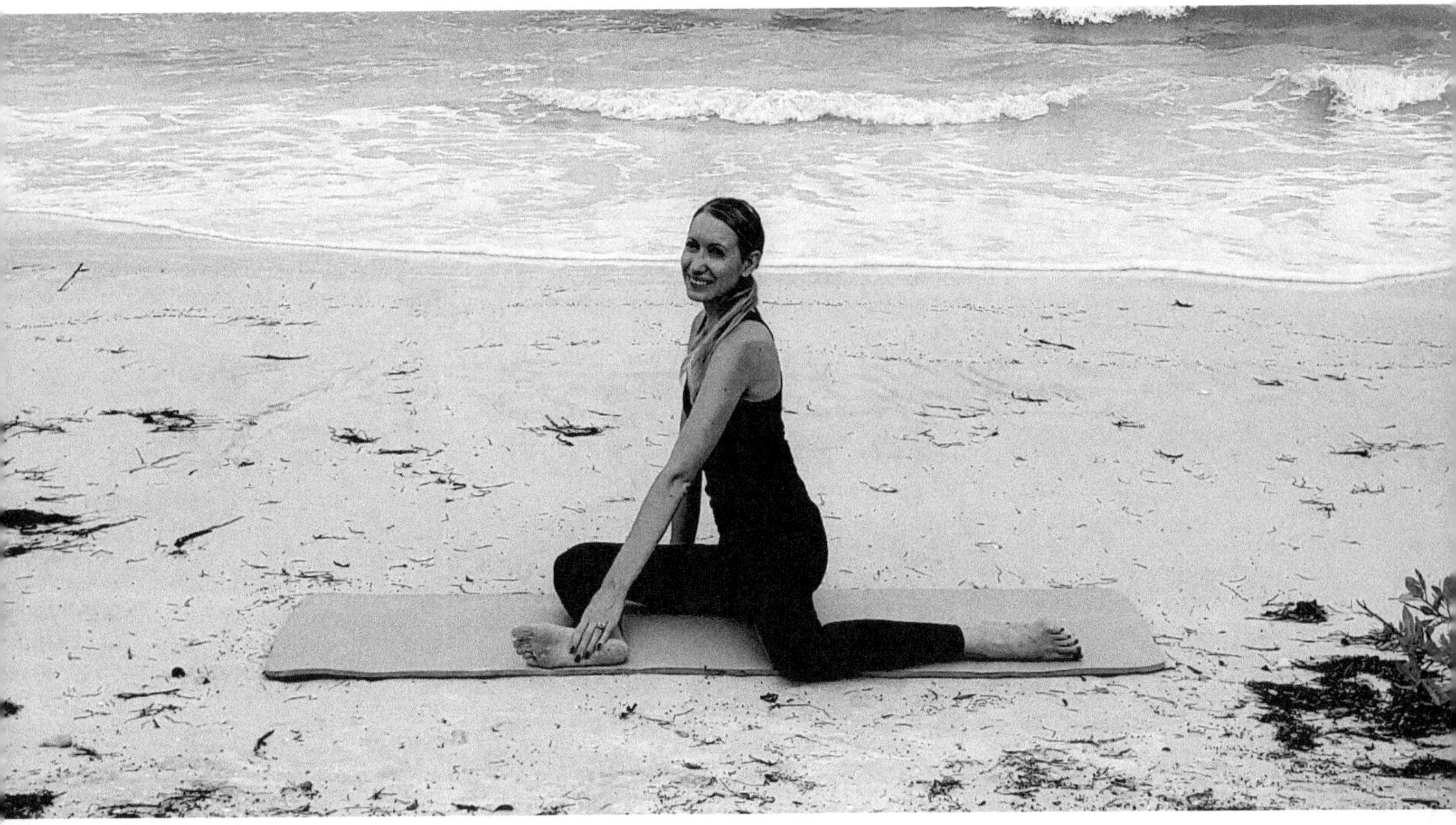

1. 90/90 Stretch - Stretches hips

2. Sit with your right knee bent at 90-degrees in front of you, calf perpendicular to your body and the sole of your foot facing to the left. Keep your right foot flexed.

3. Let your leg rest flat on the floor.

4. Place your left knee to the left of your body, and bend the knee so that your foot faces behind you. Keep your left foot flexed.

5. Keep your right butt cheek on the floor. Try to move the left cheek as close to the floor as possible. It may not be possible if you're super tight.

6. Hold for 30 seconds to 2 minutes.

7. Repeat on the other side.

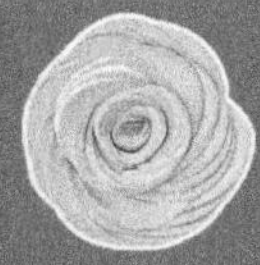

How to do Frog Stretch

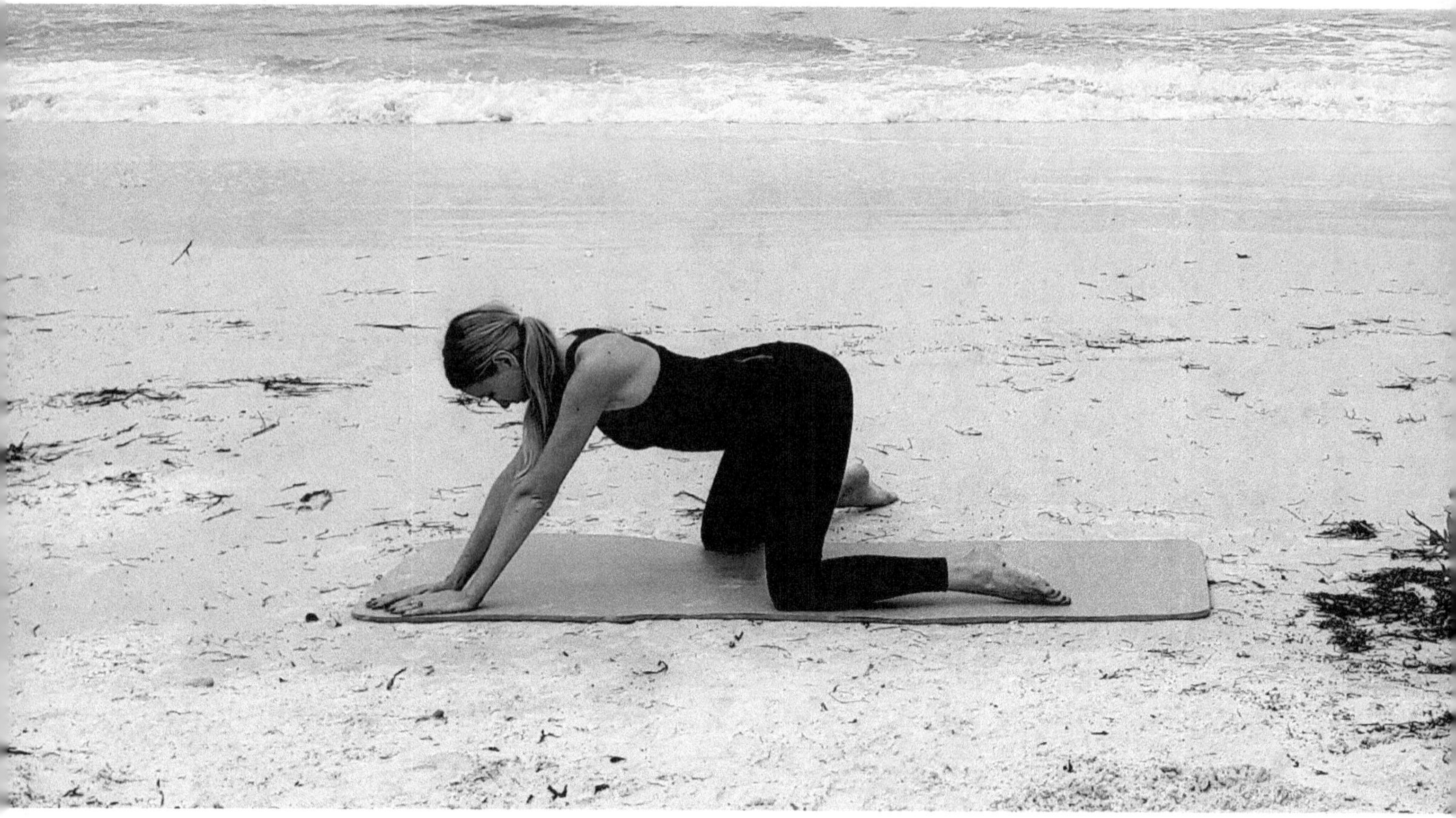

1. *Start on all fours.*

2. *Slide your knees wider than shoulder-width apart.*

3. *Turn your toes out and rest the inner edges of your feet flat on the floor.*

4. *Shift your hips back toward your heels.*

5. *Move from your hands to your forearms to get a deeper stretch, if possible.*

6. *Hold for 30 seconds to 2 minutes.*

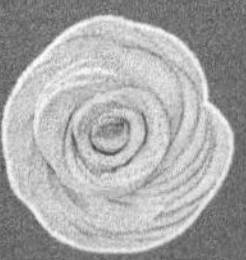

How to do Butterfly Stretch

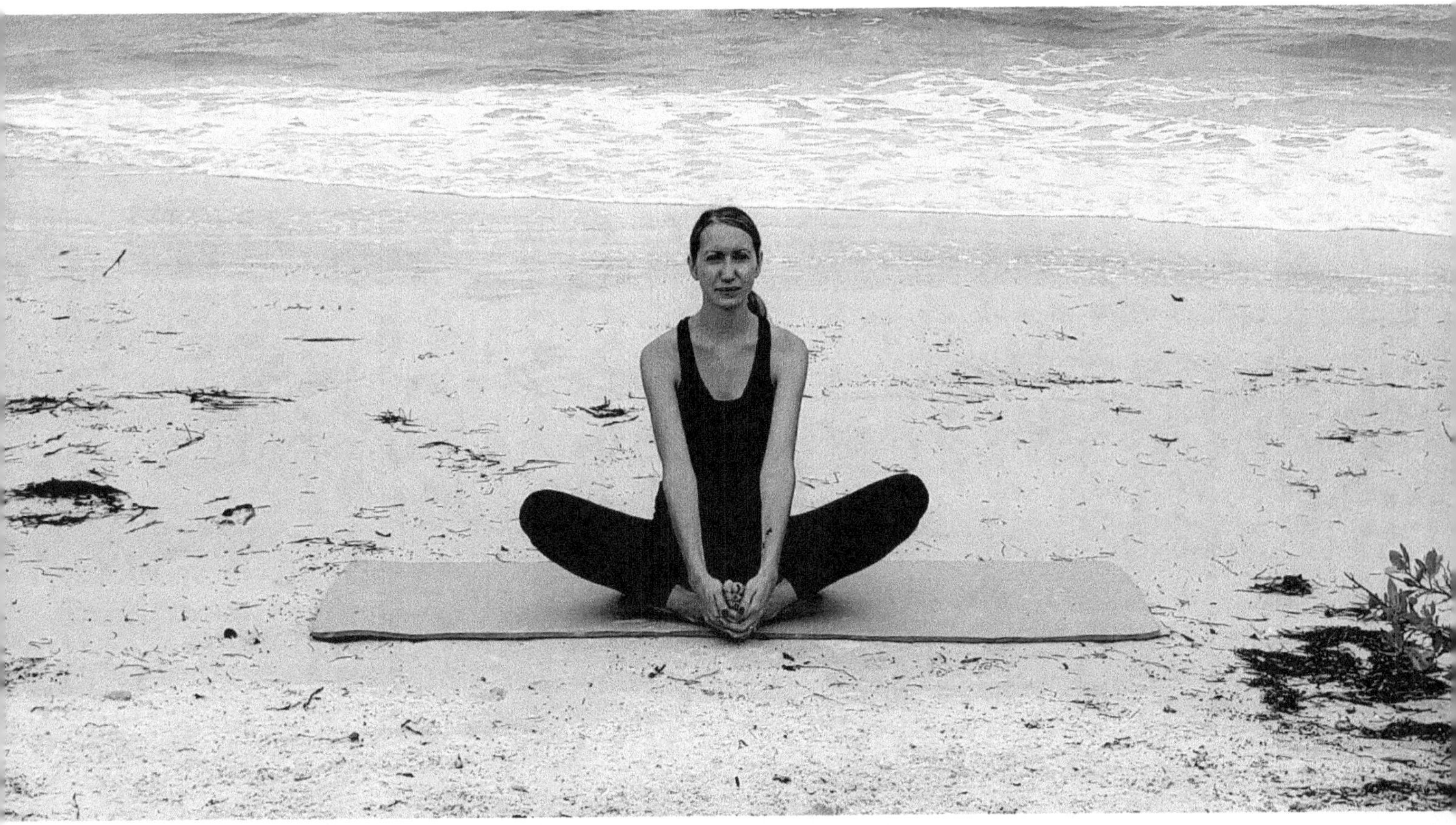

Butterfly Stretch - Stretches hips, glutes, back, thighs

1. *Sit tall on the floor with the soles of your feet together, knees bent out to sides.*

2. *Hold onto your ankles or feet, engage your abs, and slowly lower your body toward your feet as far as you can while pressing your knees toward the floor.*

3. *If you're too tight to bend over, simply press your knees down.*

4. *Hold this stretch for 30 seconds to 2 minutes.*

How to do Seated Shoulder Squeeze

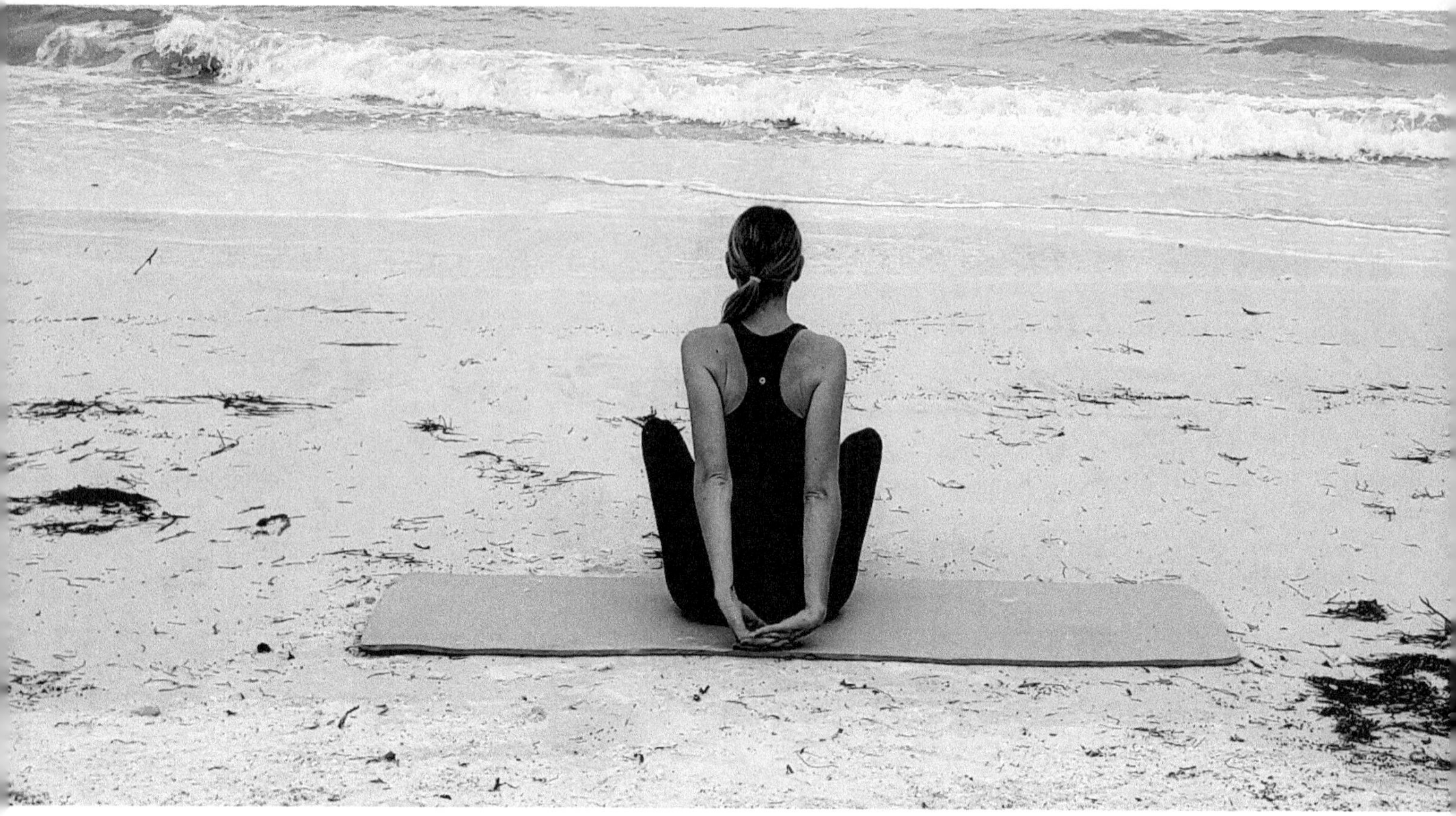

1. Sit on the floor with your knees bent and feet flat on the floor.

2. Clasp your hands behind your lower back.

3. Straighten and extend your arms and squeeze your shoulder blades together.

4. Do this for 3 seconds, and then release. Repeat 5 to 10 times.

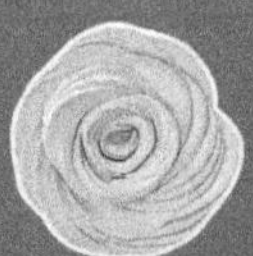

How to do Side Bend Stretch

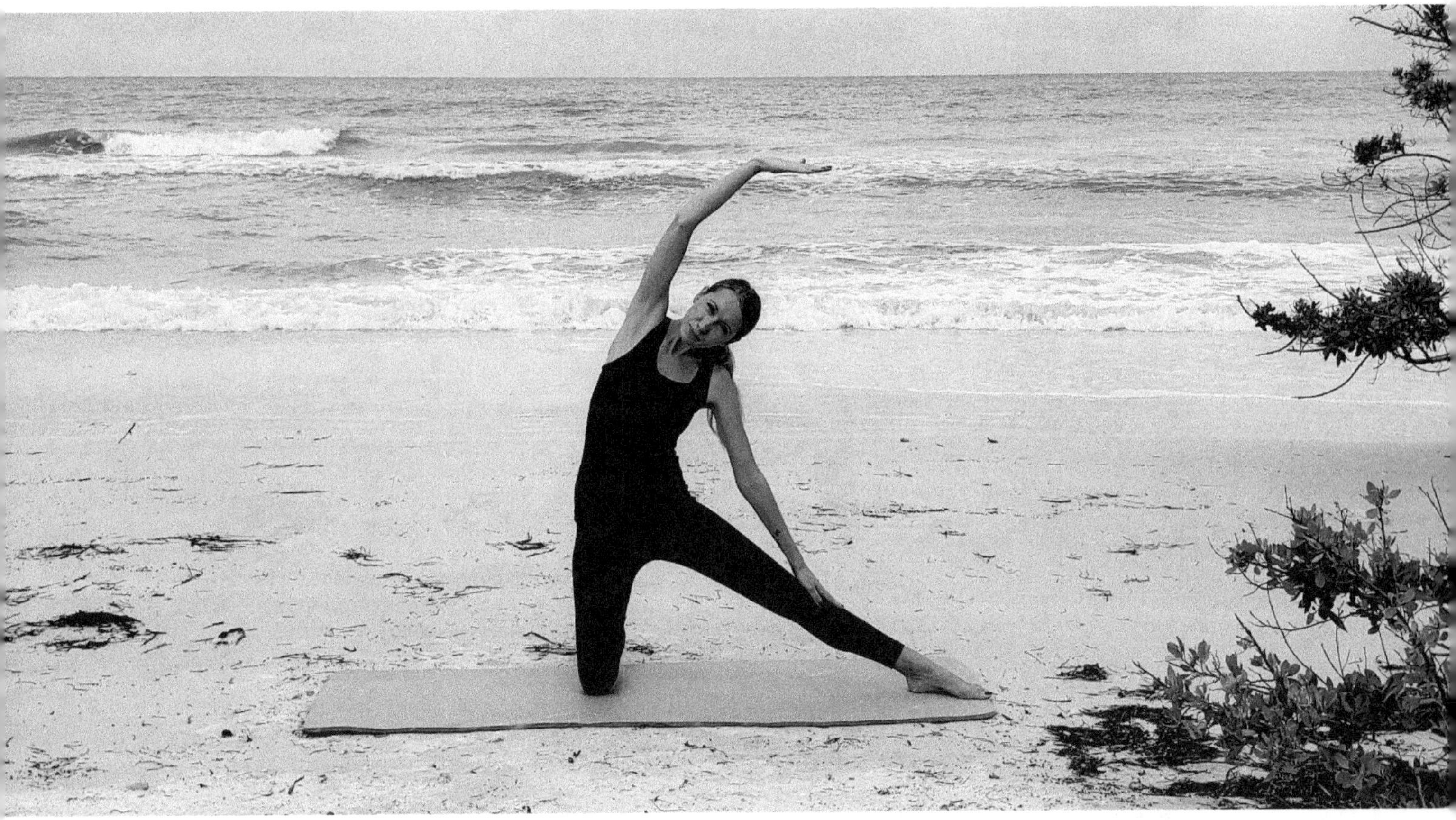

Side Bend Stretch - Stretches groin, hips, inner thigh, obliques

1. *Kneel on the floor with your legs together, back straight, and core tight.*

2. *Extend your left leg out to the side. Keep it perpendicular to your body (not in front or behind you).*

3. *Extend your right arm overhead, rest your left arm on your left leg, and gently bend your torso and right arm to the left side.*

4. *Keep your hips facing forward.*

5. *Hold this stretch for 30 seconds to 2 minutes.*

6. *Repeat on the other side.*

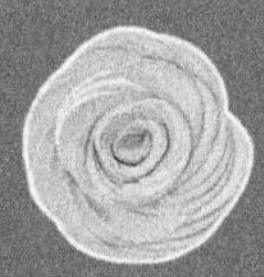

How to do Lunging Hip Flexor Stretch

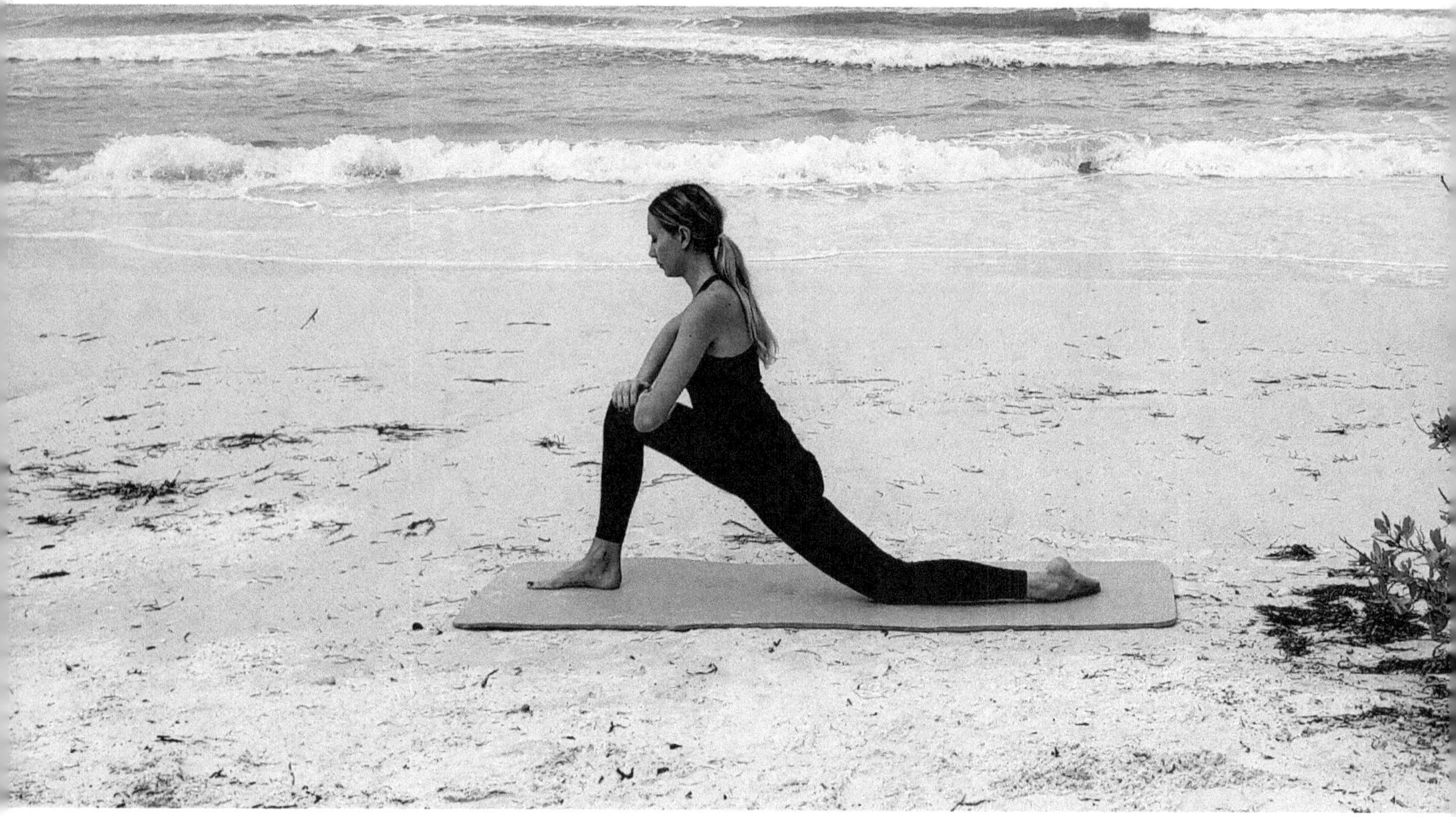

Lunging Hip Flexor Stretch - Stretches hips, quads, glutes

1. *Kneel on your left knee. Place your right foot flat on the floor in front of you, knee bent.*

2. *Lean forward, stretching your left hip toward the floor.*

3. *Squeeze your butt; this will allow you to stretch your hip flexor even more.*

4. *Hold for 30 seconds to 2 minutes.*

5. *Switch sides and repeat.*

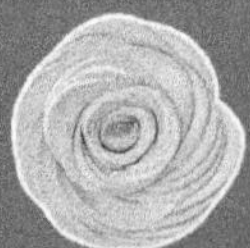

How to do Lying Pectoral Stretch

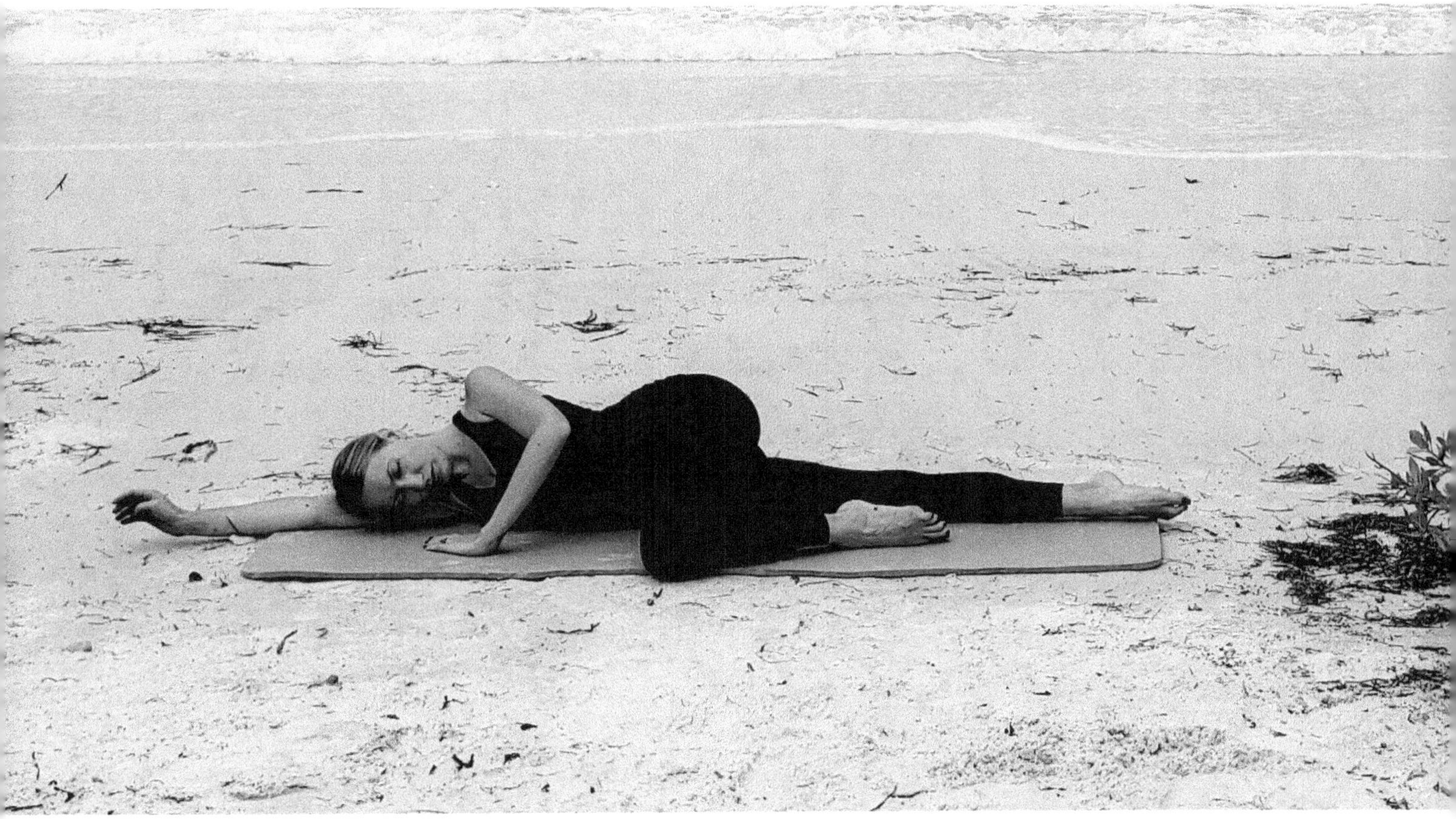

Lying Pectoral Stretch - Stretches chest, shoulders

1. *Lie on your stomach with both arms extended to the sides so your body is in a T shape.*

2. *Push off the ground with your left hand and bend your left knee for balance as you start to roll to your right side. You should feel this in your right-side pectoral muscles.*

3. *As your mobility increases, you'll be able to stretch further and roll your body further.*

4. *Repeat on the other side.*

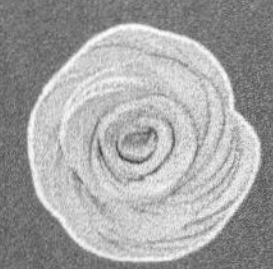

How to do Knee to Chest Stretch

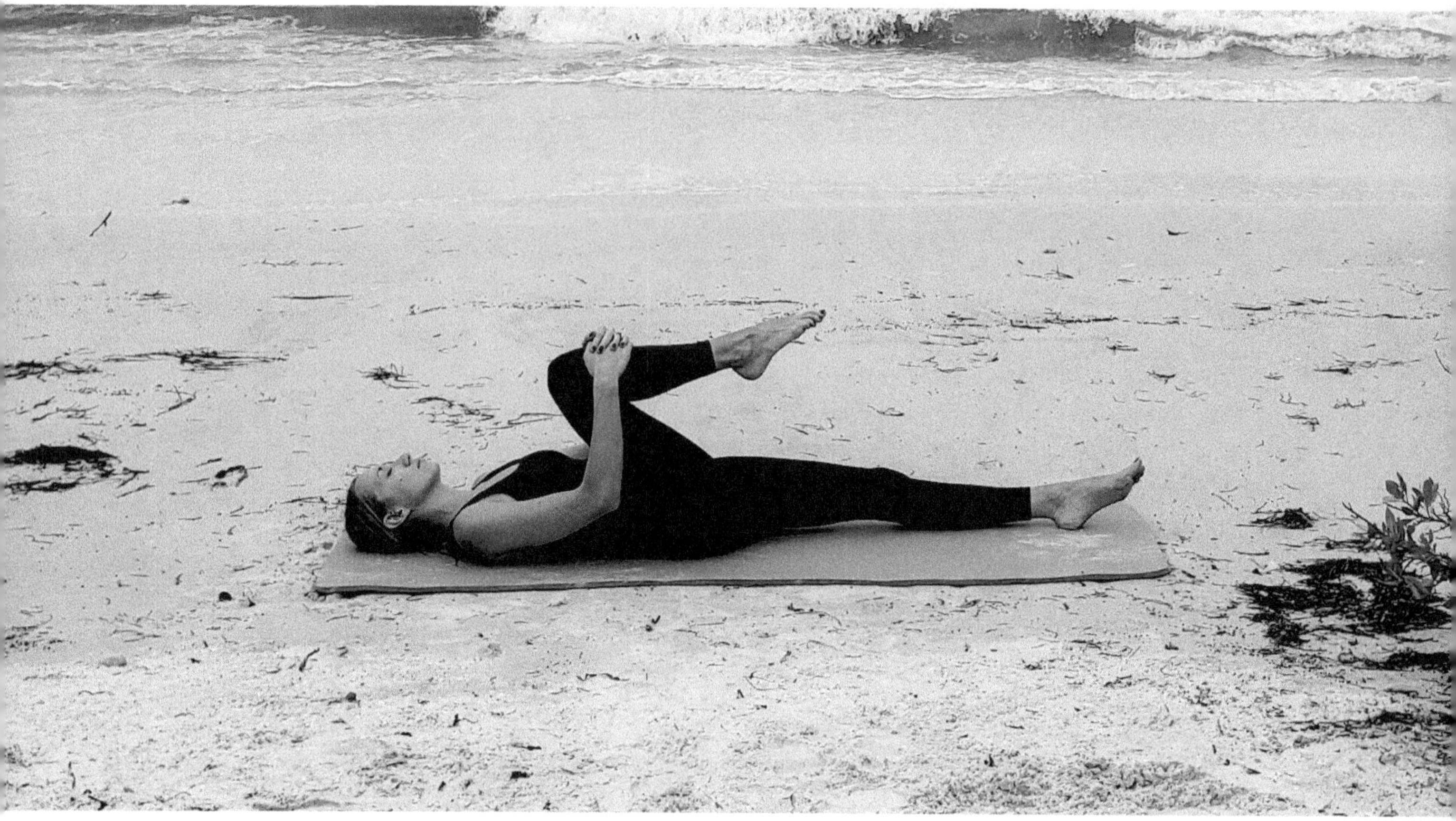

Knee to Chest Stretch - Stretches lower back, hips, hamstrings

1. Lie on your back with both legs extended.

2. Pull your right knee into your chest, while keeping the left leg straight and your lower back pressed into the floor.

3. Hold for 30 seconds to 2 minutes.

4. Repeat on the other leg.

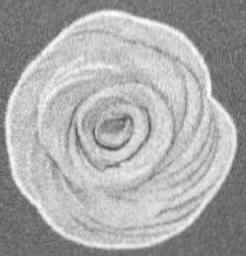

How to do Seated Neck Release

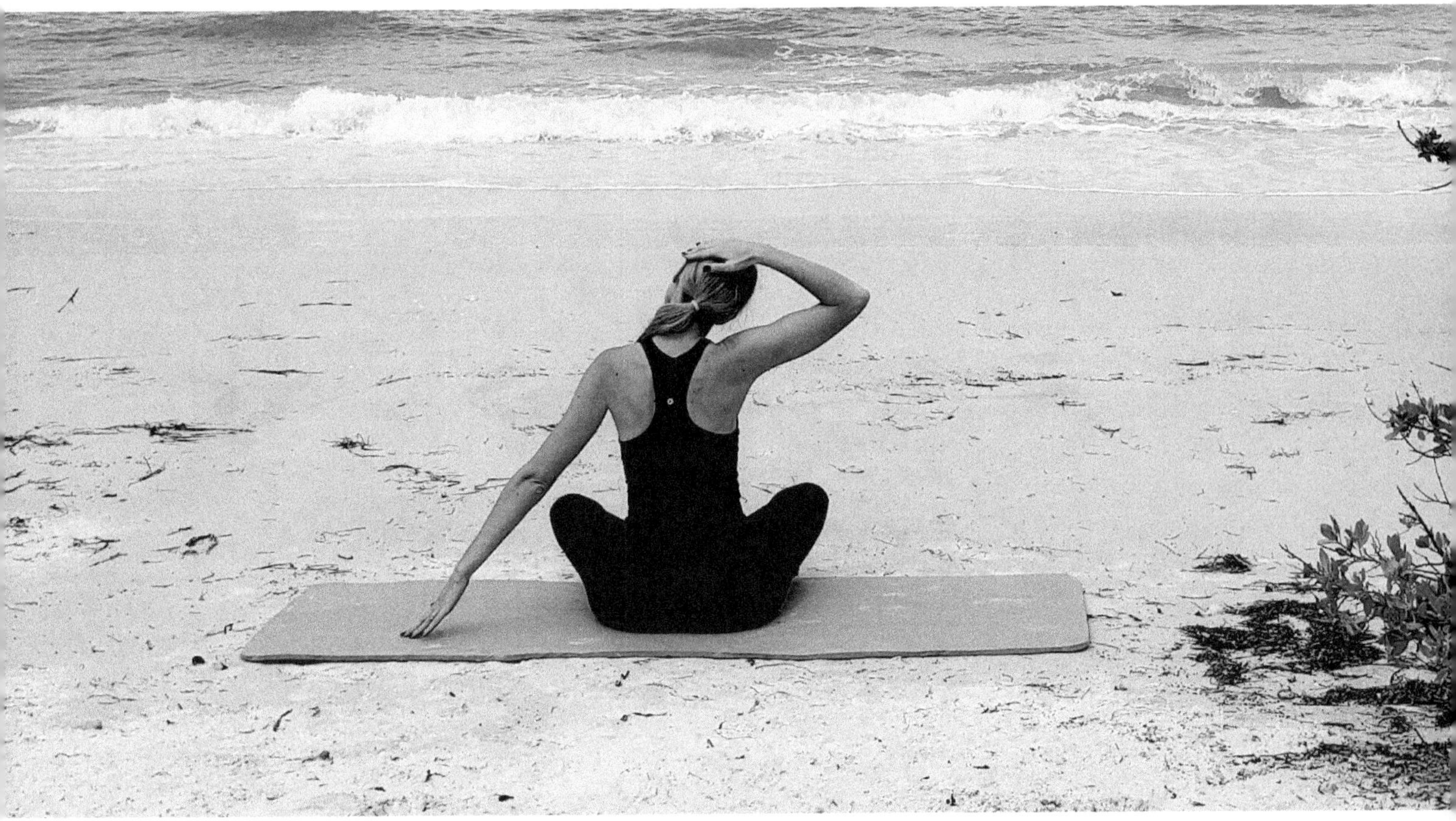

Seated Neck Release - Stretches neck

1. *Stand with feet shoulder-width apart, or sit down with your back straight and chest lifted.*

2. *Drop your left ear to your left shoulder.*

3. *To deepen the stretch, gently press down on your head with your left hand.*

4. *Hold for 30 seconds to 2 minutes.*

5. *Switch to repeat on opposite side.*

How to do Lying Quad Stretch

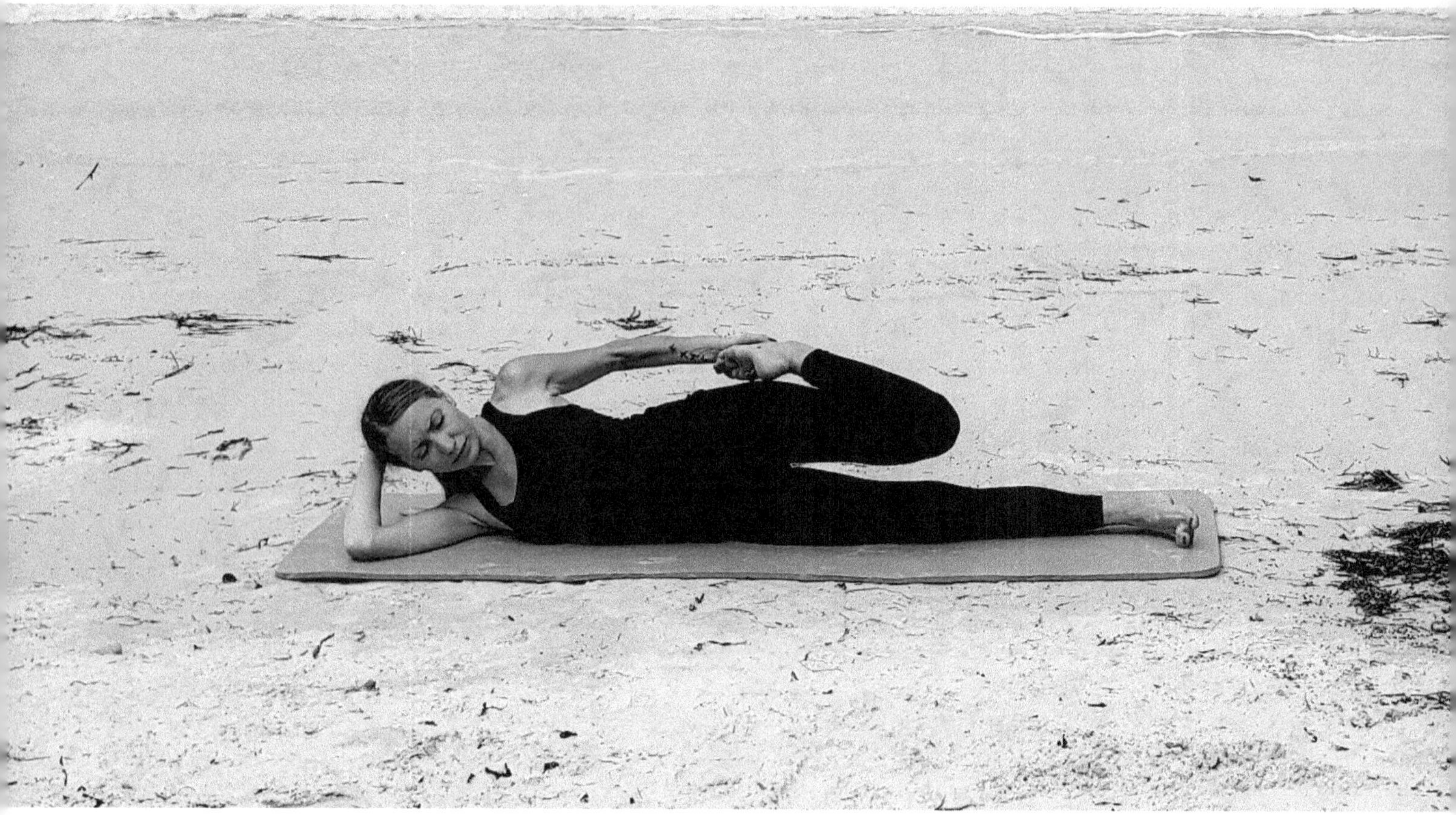

Lying Quad Stretch - Stretches quads

1. *Lie on one side.*

2. *Keep your bottom leg straight and bend your top knee so your foot is by your butt.*

3. *Hold your top foot with your hand, pulling it toward your butt.*

4. *Keep your hips stable so you're not rocking back as you pull.*

5. *Hold for 30 seconds to 2 minutes.*

6. *Switch sides and repeat.*

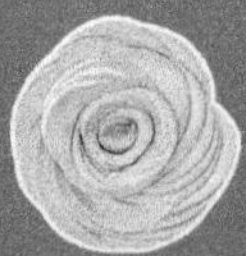

How to do Sphinx Pose

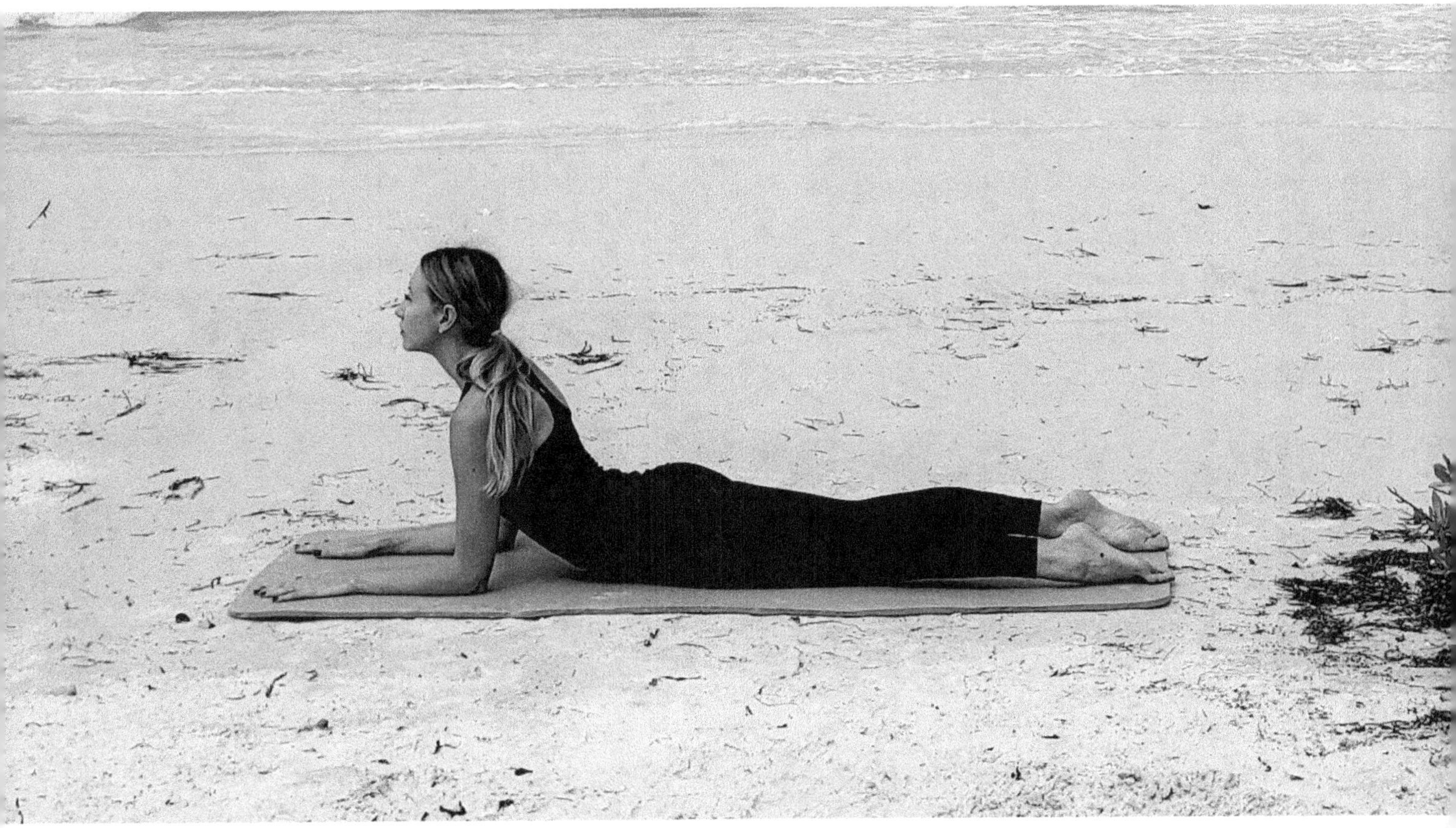

Sphinx Pose - Stretches lower back, chest, shoulders

1. *Lie on your stomach with your legs straight out behind you.*

2. *Place your elbows under your shoulders and your forearms on the floor as you lift your chest up off the floor.*

3. *Press your hips and thighs into the floor, and think about lengthening your spine while keeping your shoulders relaxed.*

4. *Sit up just enough to feel a nice stretch in your lower back. Don't hyperextend, and stop immediately if you start to feel any discomfort or pain.*

How to do Extended Puppy Pose

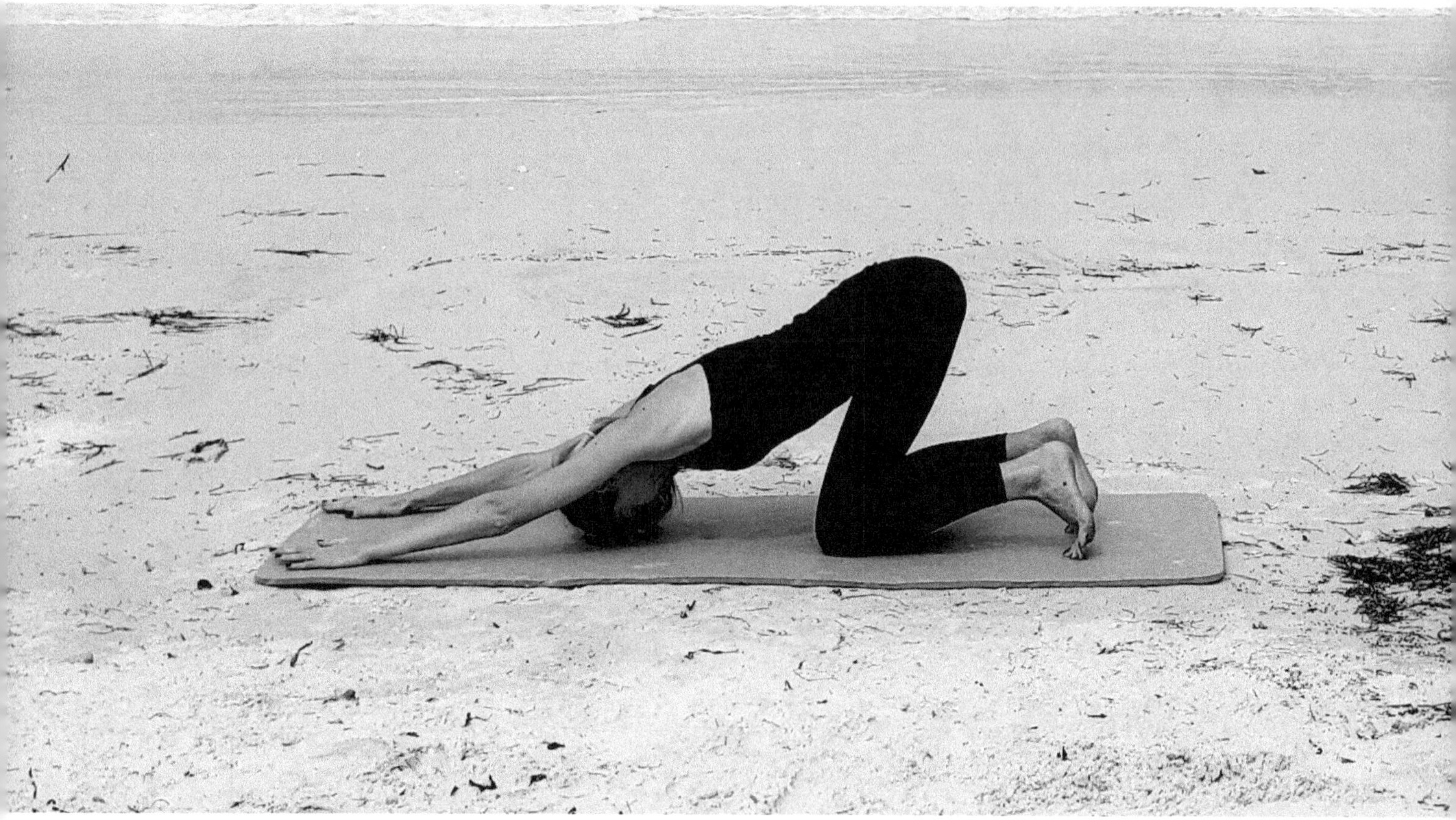

Extended Puppy Pose - Stretches back, shoulders, glutes

1. *Start on all fours.*

2. *Walk your arms forward a few inches and curl your toes under.*

3. *Push your hips up and back halfway toward your heels.*

4. *Push through the palms of your hands to keep your arms straight and engaged.*

5. *Hold for 30 seconds to 2 minutes.*

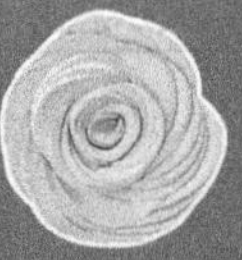

How to do Reclining Bound Angle Pose

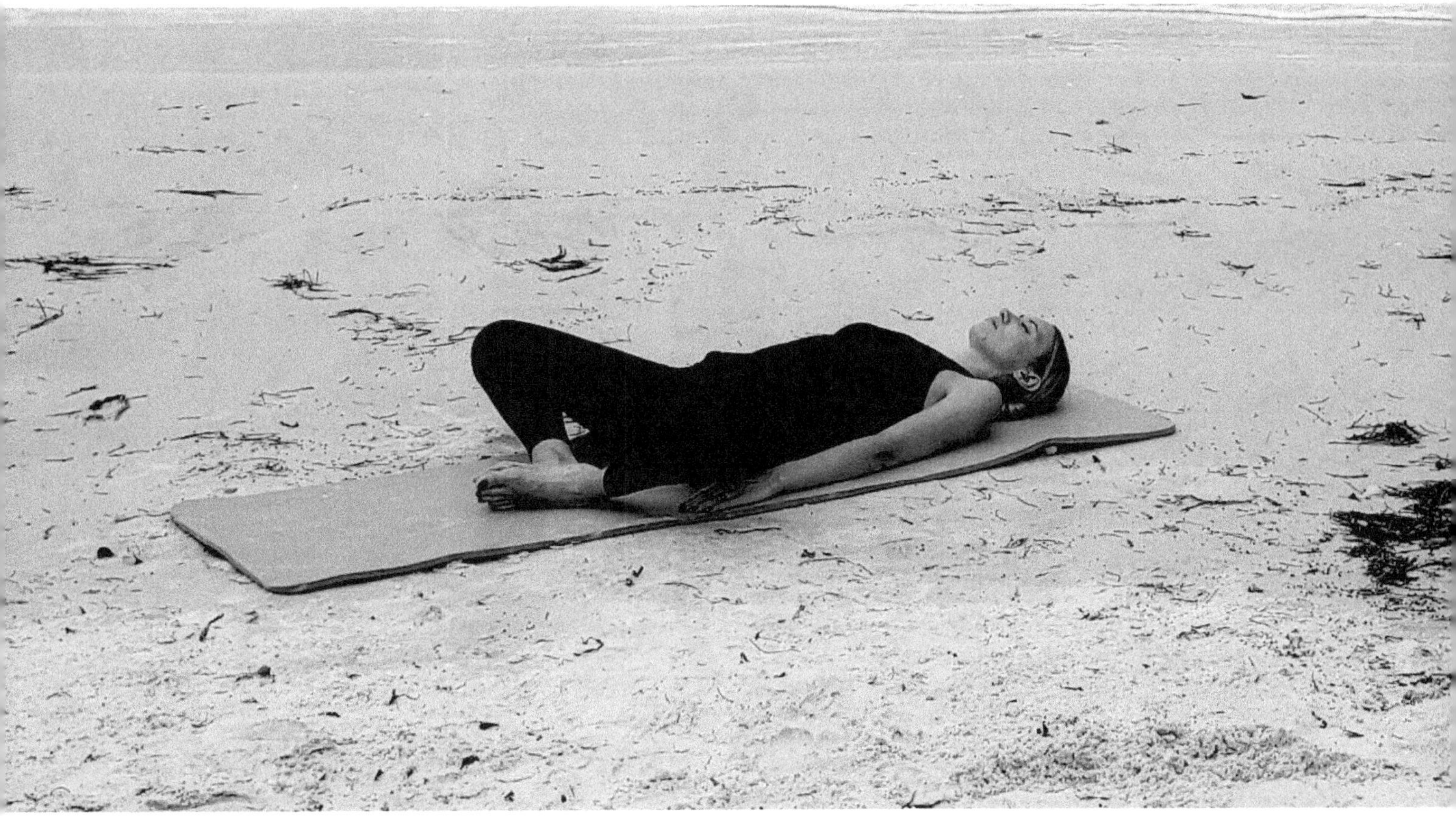

Reclining Bound Angle Pose - Stretches inner thighs, hips, groin

1. *Lie on your back.*

2. *Bring the soles of your feet together and allow your knees to open up and move closer to the floor.*

3. *Hold for 30 seconds to 2 minutes.*

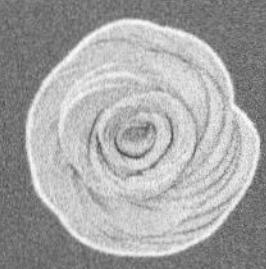

How to do Standing Quad Stretch

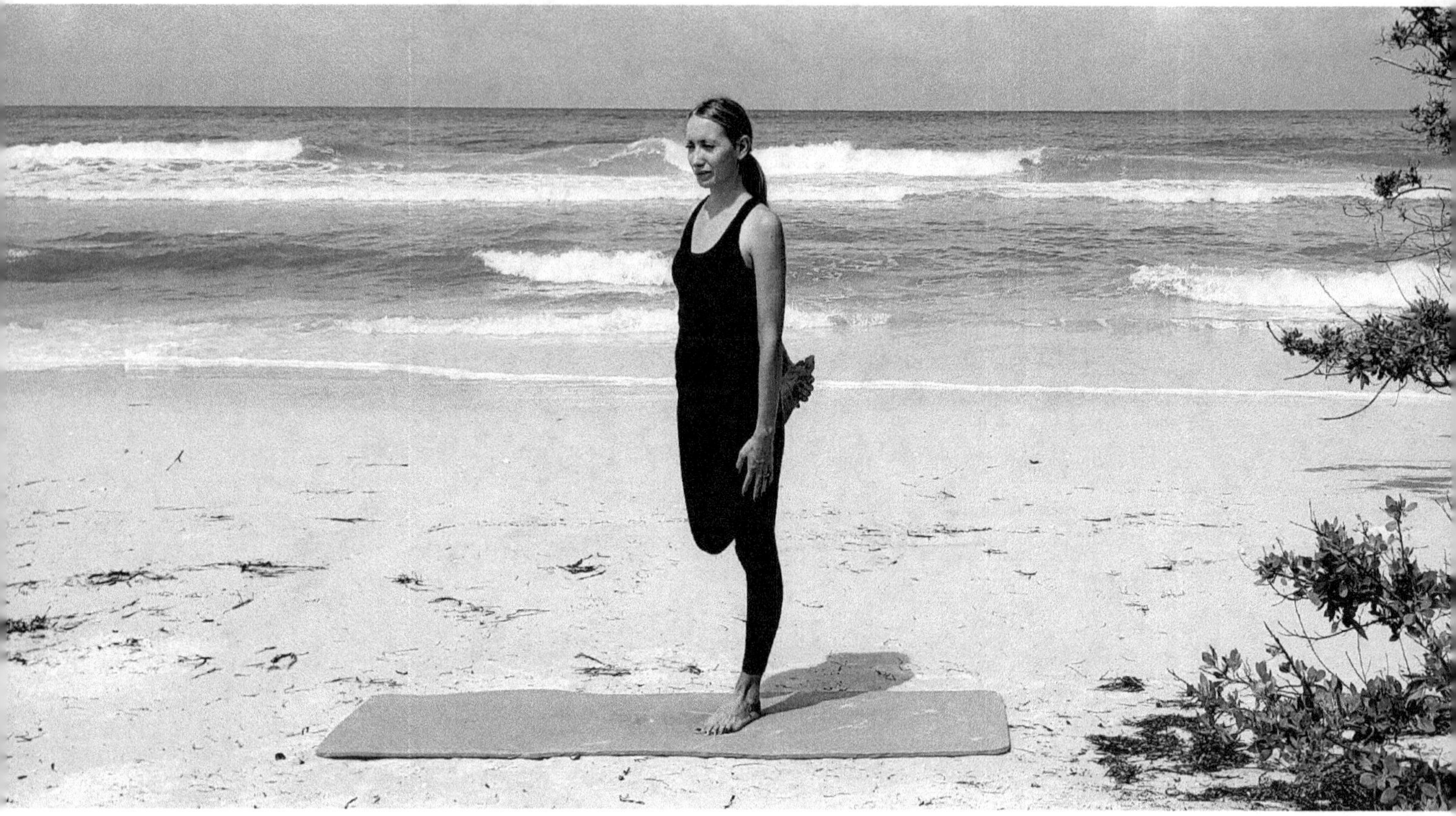

Standing Quad Stretch - Stretches quads

1. Stand with your feet together.

2. Bend your left knee and use your left hand to pull your left foot toward your butt. Keep your knees together.
   (If you need to, put one hand on a wall for balance.)

3. Squeeze your glutes to increase the stretch in the front of your legs.

4. Hold for 30 seconds to 2 minutes.

5. Repeat on the other leg.

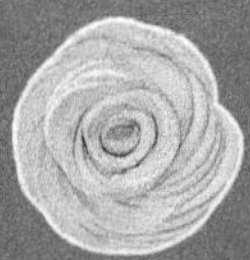

How to do Knees to Chest

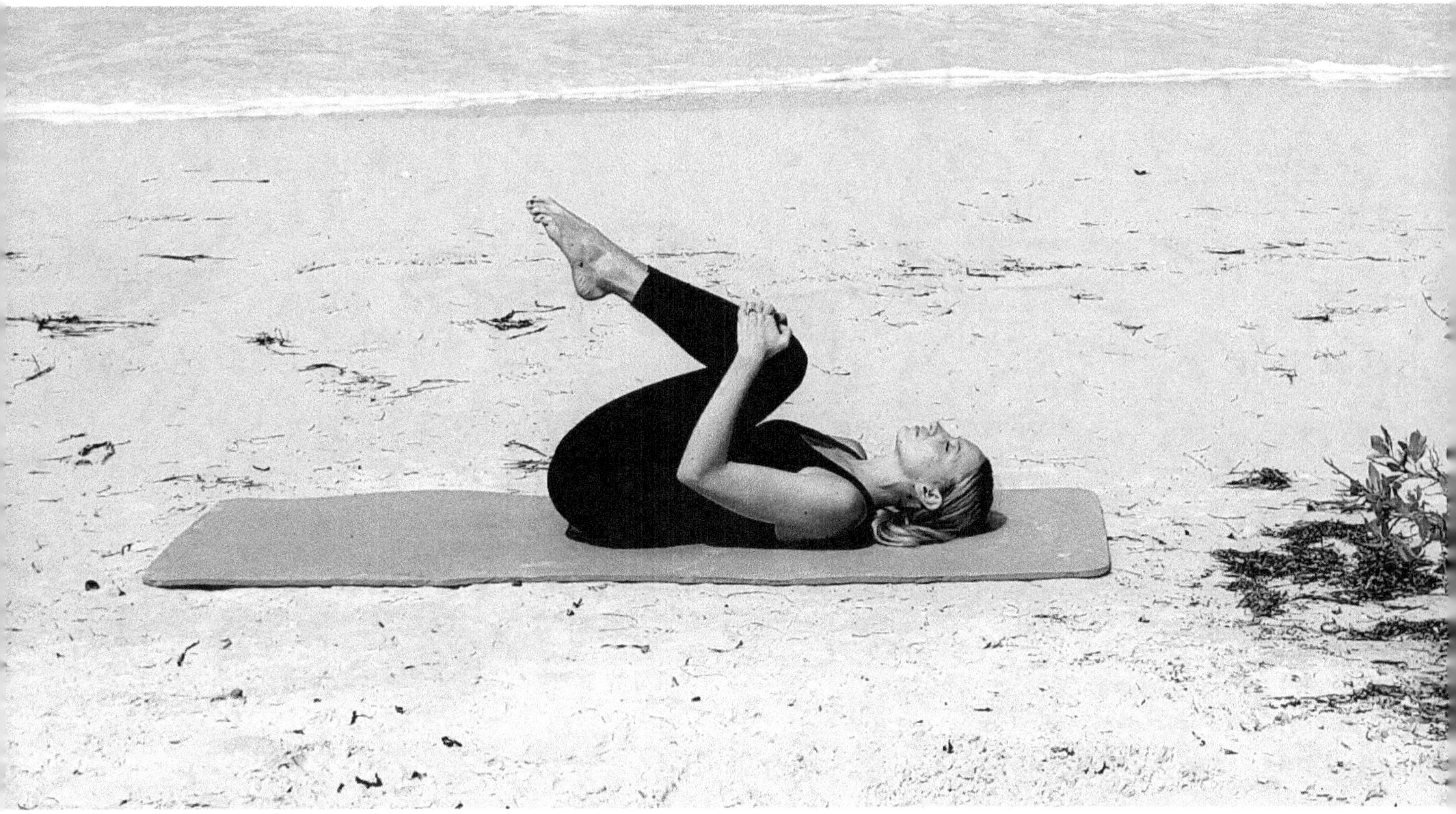

Knees to Chest - Stretches lower back, glutes

1. Lie on your back and pull your knees into your chest with both hands.

2. Keep your lower back on the floor.

3. Hold for 30 seconds to 2 minutes.

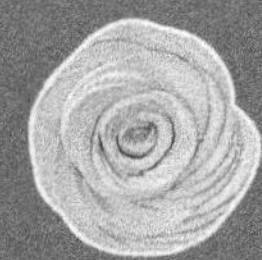

How to do Cat-camel back stretch

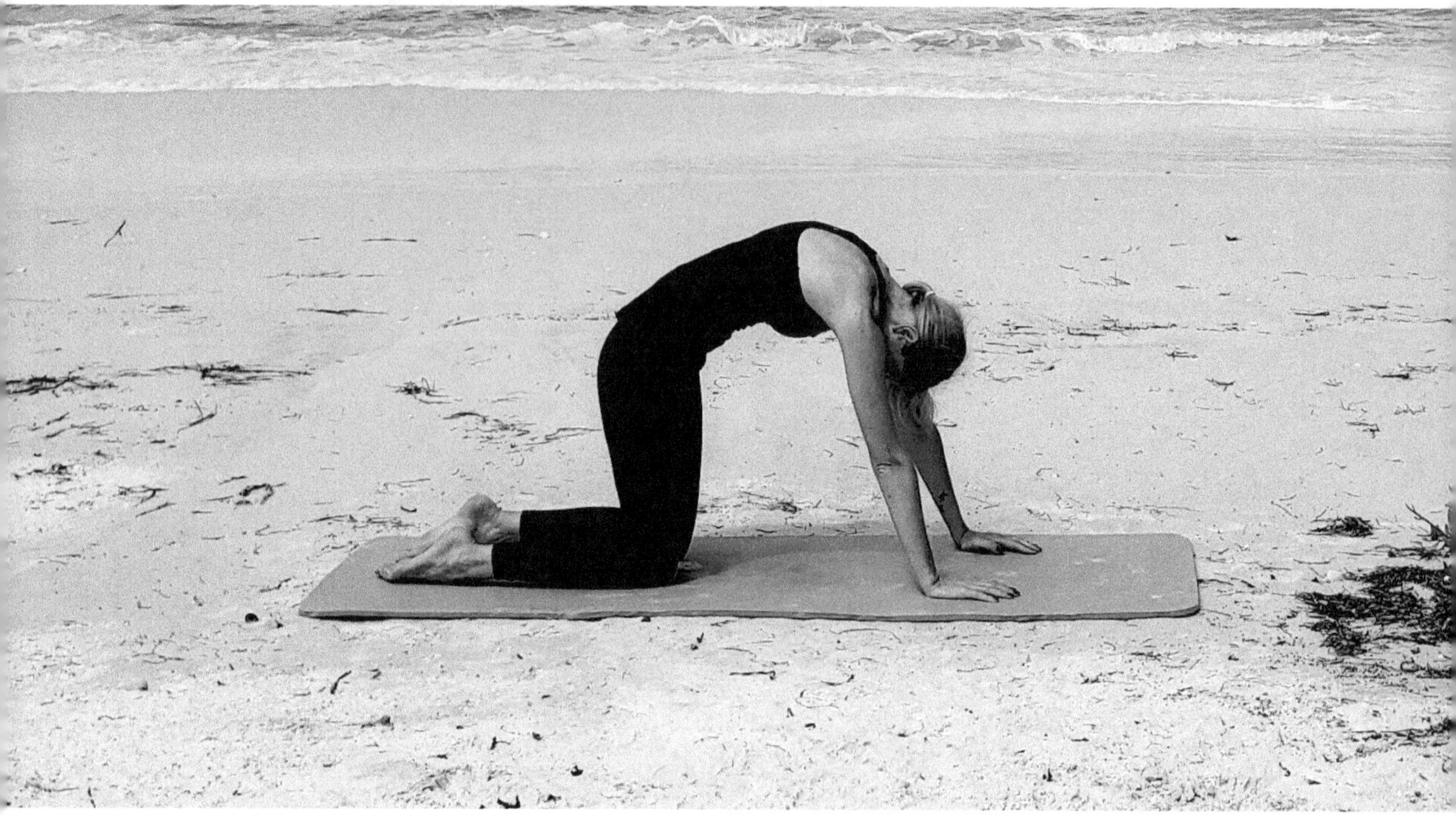

1. *Get onto your hands and knees.*

2. *Slowly alternate between arching and rounding your back upwards so that all three sections of your lower, middle, and upper spine are extended together. Do this slowly and gently.*

3. *Do one stretch up to three to four seconds.*

4. *Repeat stretch five or six times.*

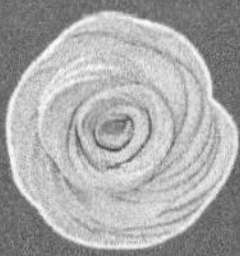

How to do Seated forward bend

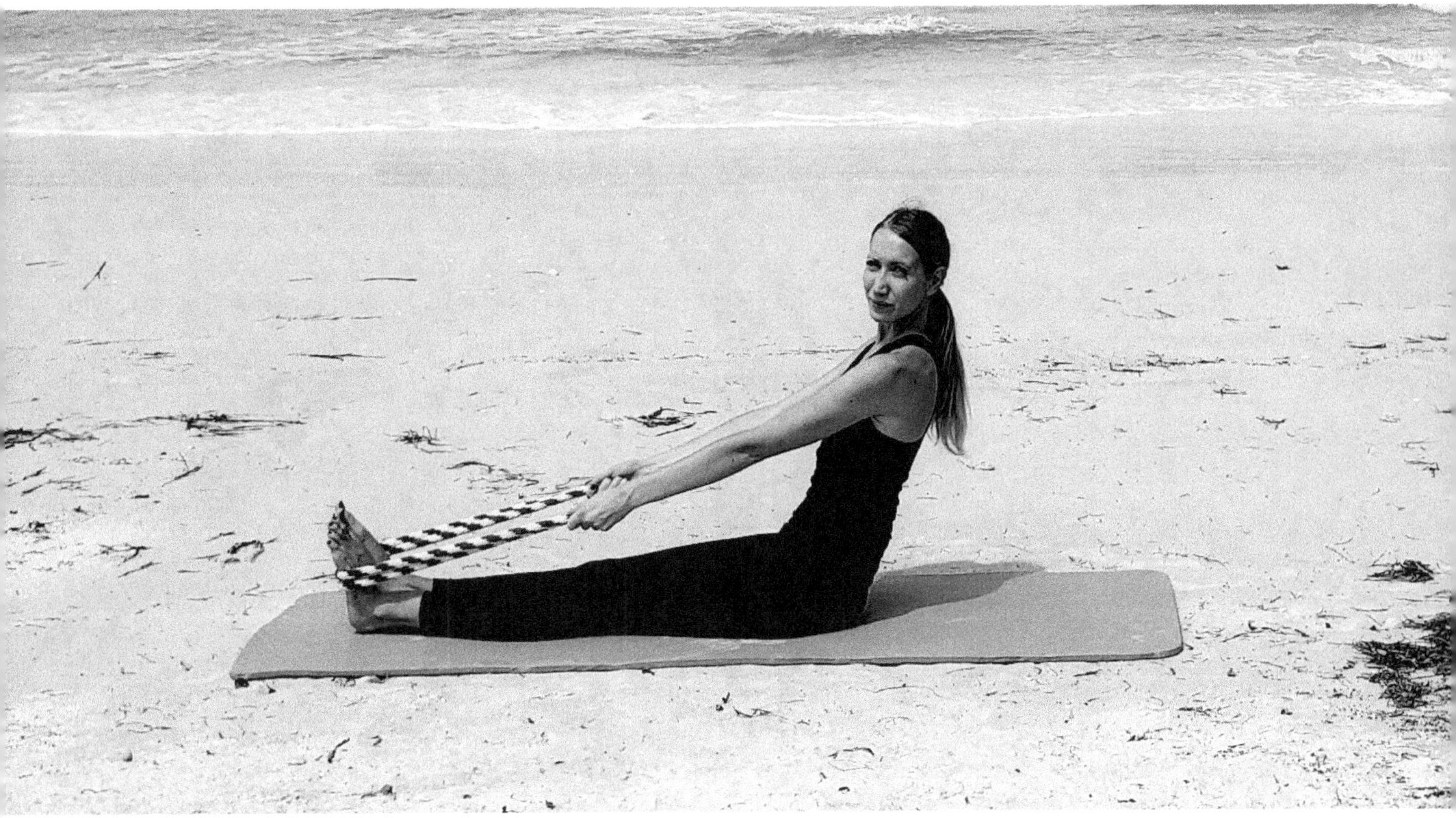

1. *Sit on the floor with your legs straight out in front of you.*

2. *Hook a yoga strap rope or towel around the bottom of your feet, and leave it there for now.*

3. *Inhale and reach your arms up to the ceiling.*

4. *Exhale and begin to bend forward gently by hinging at the hips, and bring your belly down to your thighs.*

5. *Grasp the yoga strap rope or towel, keeping your back straight. You want to lengthen the spine and keep your neck in line with your body.*

6. *Take another breath and, as you exhale, see if you can bring your upper body even closer to your legs.*

7. *Hold for between 30 seconds and three minutes.*

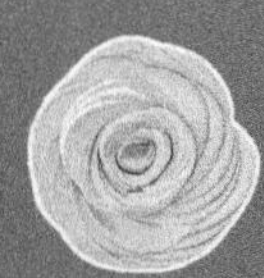

How to do Side Stretch

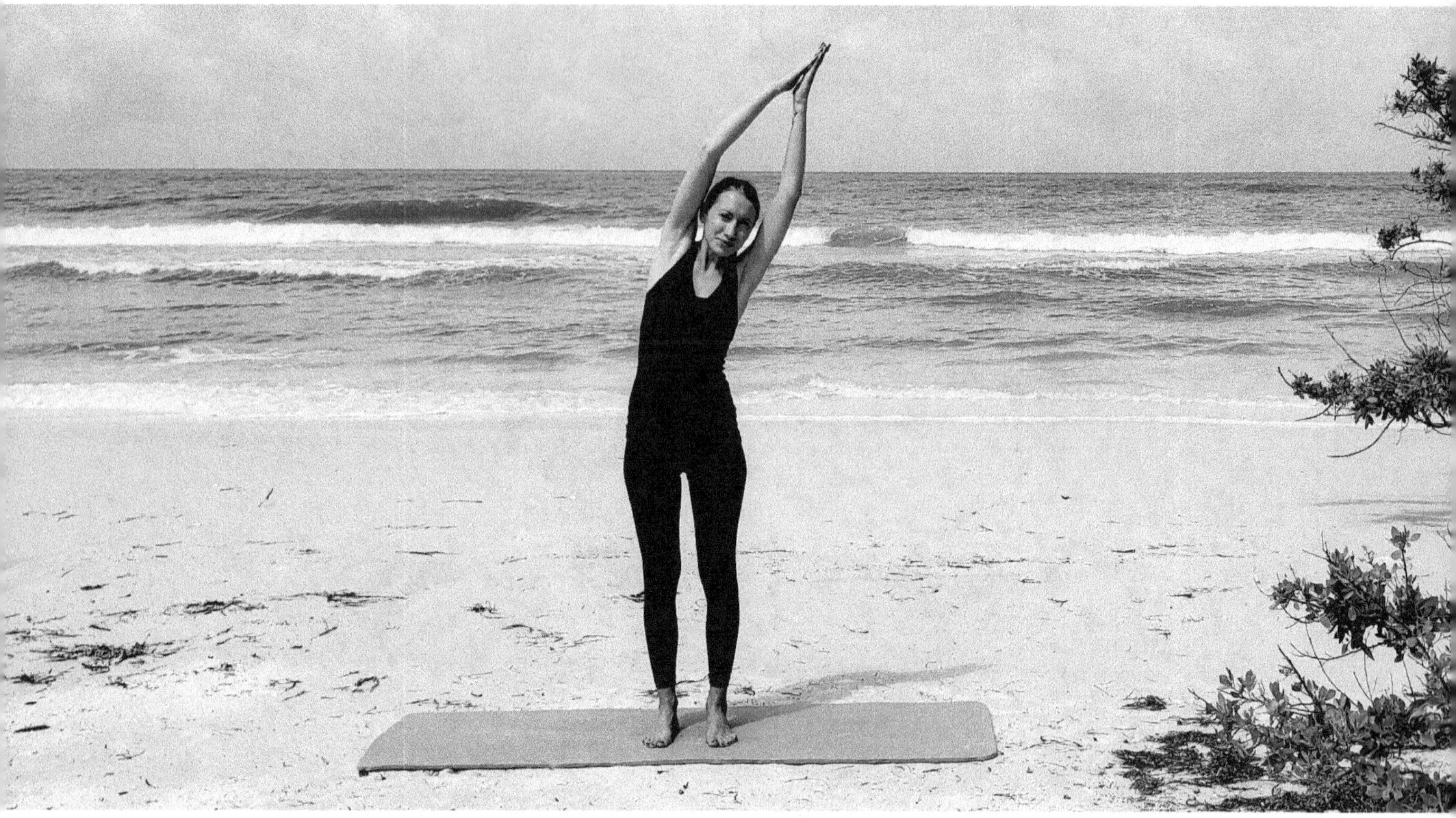

1. *Raise your arms straight above you and clasp your hands together.*

2. *Push your hands up and then over to each side of you.*

www.ketoveo.com

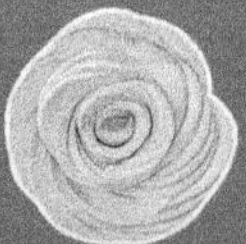

How to do Standing Rolls

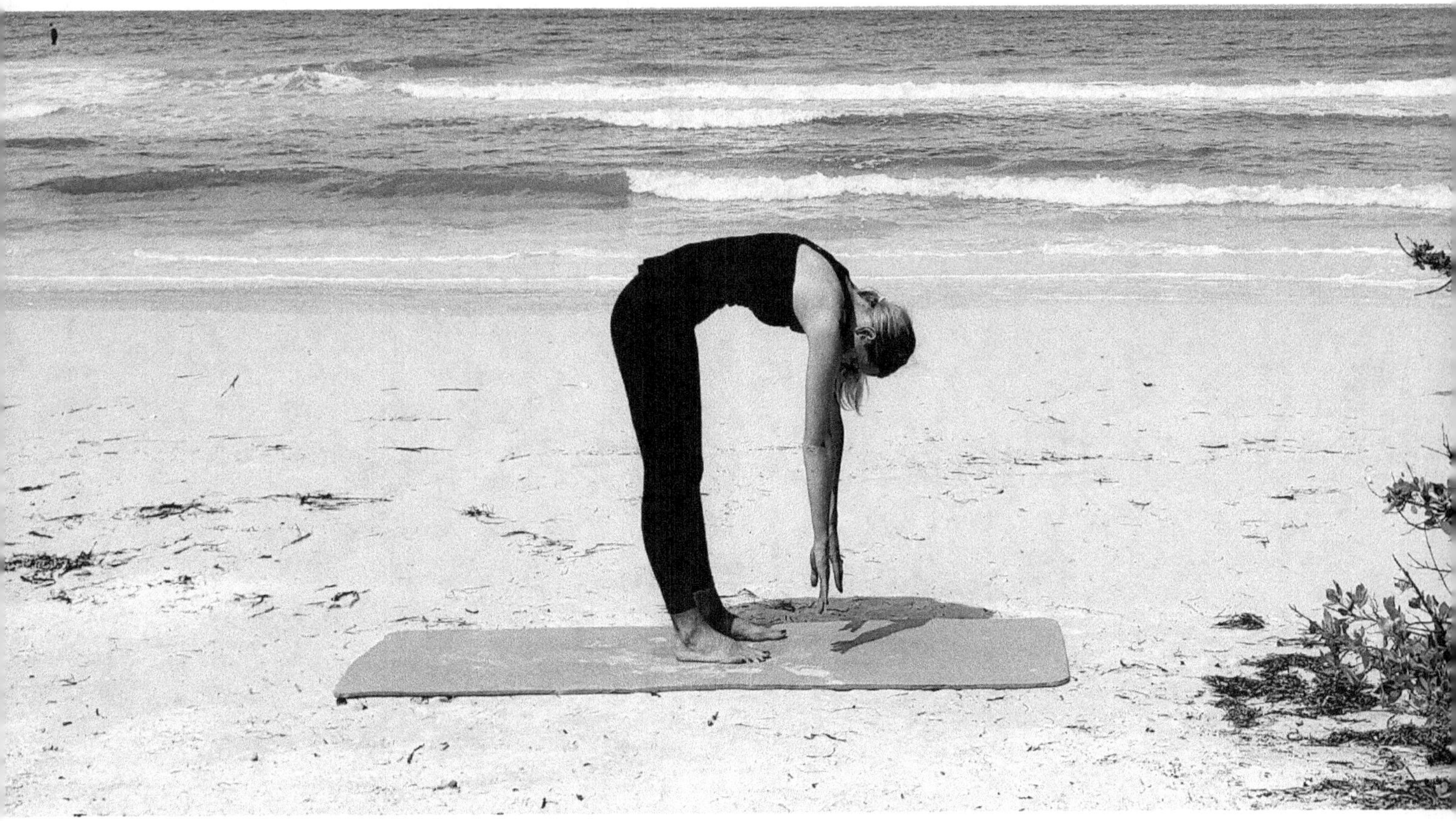

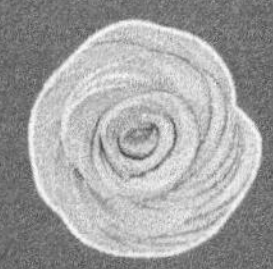

1. *Begin standing parallel hips width apart, knees soft.*

2. *Inhale and lower your chin towards your chest.*

3. *Exhaling while bending your head, shoulders, chest, and upper torso until you are unable to bend any further.*

4. *Inhale filling your ribcage, whilst being paused at the bottom, standing firmly on both feet, knees soft and not locked.*

5. *Exhale and slowly pull yourself up by pulling your navel up to your spine as you stack your pelvis and vertebrae one on top of the other with your head coming up last.*

6. *Repeat 3-5 times.*

How to do Upper Back Stretch

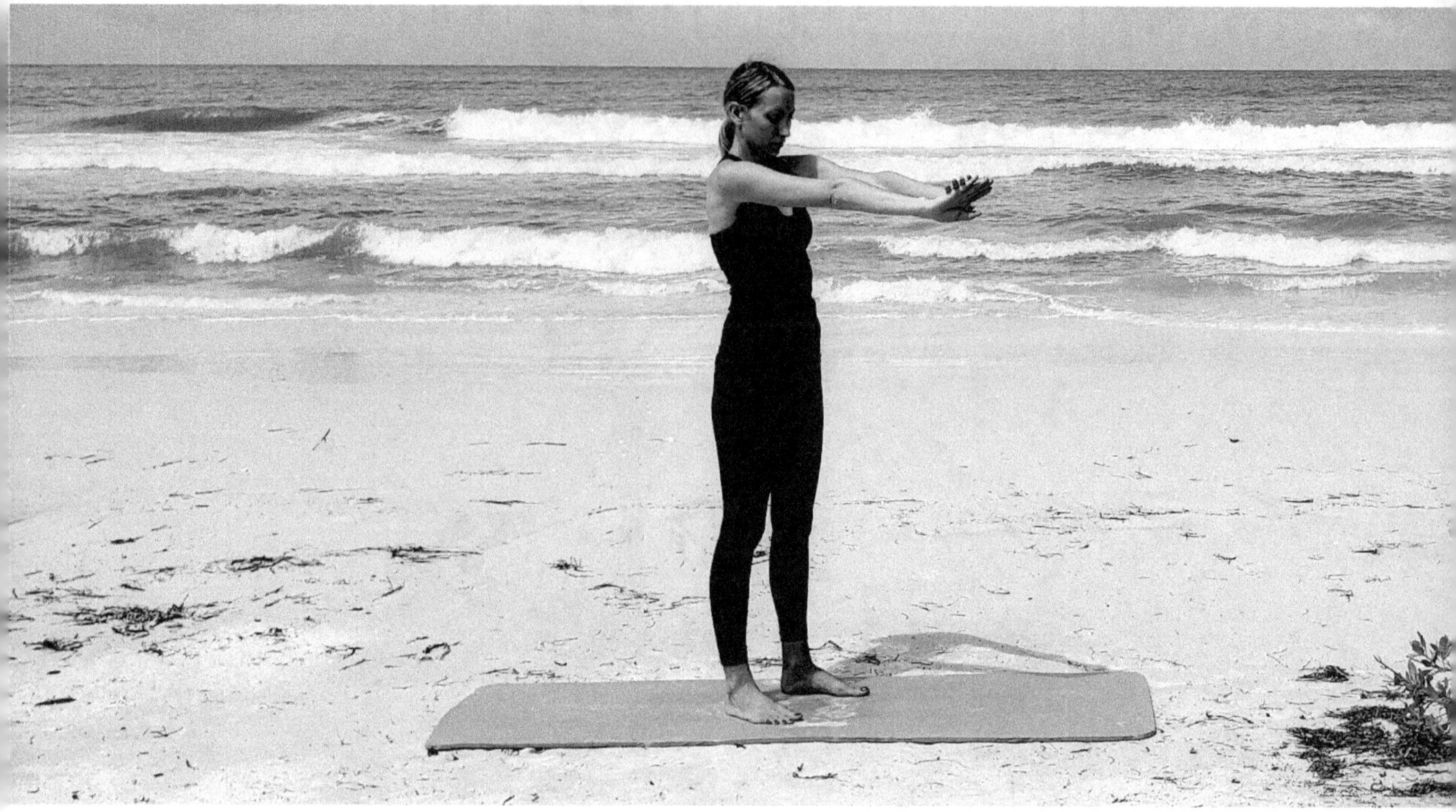

1. Stand up straight or sit on a surface so that your legs are at a 90 degree angle.

2. Place one hand on top of the other with arms straight in front of you.

3. Press your arms away from your body.

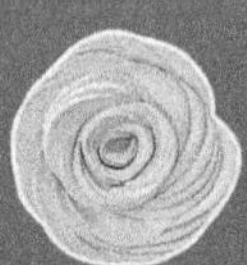

www.ingramcontent.com/pod-product-compliance
Lightning Source LLC
Chambersburg PA
CBHW081019260726
48662CB00025B/2464